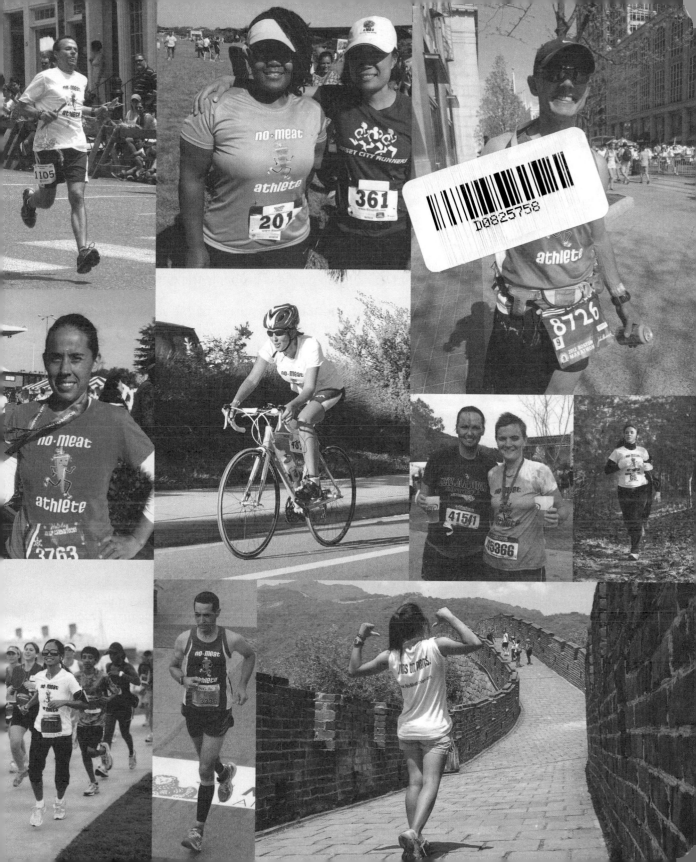

"*No Meat Athlete* will not only power your strength and endurance, it will give you an extra edge in every aspect of your life."

—**Neal Barnard, M.D.**, author of *Power Foods for the Brain*

"As a runner who began competing in the days of the traditional steak training meal, I welcome this book's enlightening confirmation of my own experience: Athletes who pass on the meat can perform at the highest level and still enjoy their meals to the max. "

—**Ed Ayres**, founder, *Running Times* magazine, and author of *The Longest Race: A Lifelong Runner, an Iconic Ultramarathon, and the Case for Human Endurance*

"Matt Frazier is a rising star in the world of vegan athletes. Covering the mechanics of diet and training as well as the transformative nature of a whole-foods, plant-based diet, he demonstrates that a body running on plants is probably the one ahead of you at the finish line!"

—**Colleen Patrick-Goudreau**, author of *The Vegan Table* and *The Joy of Vegan Baking*

"Anyone can become a no meat athlete, and Matt Frazier provides the roadmap to wellness and performance no matter where the journey takes you."

—**Scott Jurek**, world-renowned ultramarathon champion and author of *Eat and Run*

"In this fantastic book, Matt clearly lays out a simple but powerful plan for changing your eating habits. In small steps, you can create a healthier, stronger, more compassionate diet that will fuel the best version of you."

—**Leo Babauta**, simplicity blogger at zenhabits.net

"Matt Frazier takes all the guesswork out of maximizing your health the plant-based way with his bulletproof primer *No Meat Athlete*. Whether you are an elite marathoner or a weekend warrior, this clear, concise, and no-nonsense book is your one-stop roadmap to creating and maintaining a sustainable plant-based lifestyle. All hail the running carrot!"

—**Rich Roll**, plant-based ultra-distance athlete and author of *Finding Ultra: Rejecting Middle Age, Becoming One of the World's Fittest Men, and Discovering Myself*

". . . an inspiring and empowering book for people interested in being healthy, happy, and active. I highly recommend this accessible, life-changing book."

—**Gene Baur**, founder, Farm Sanctuary

"If you've been waiting for the inspiration to turn your life around (by changing what you eat), here it is. It might not make the industrial food complex happy, but you'll be glad you did."

—**Seth Godin**, author of *The Icarus Deception*

NO LONGER PROPERTY OF
SEATTLE PUBLIC LIBRARY

"Well-organized, very accessible, and a joy to read. This book gives you the real how and why of healthy living with real-life applications, actual training plans, and easy recipes—Frazier nailed it with this book."

—**Sid Garza-Hillman**, author of *Approaching the Natural: A Health Manifesto*

". . . an excellent resource for the new or experienced athlete. If you are looking for an outstanding guide to improving your health and fitness, *No Meat Athlete* is the book for you."

—**Robert Cheeke**, author of *Vegan Bodybuilding & Fitness: The Complete Guide to Building Your Body on a Plant-Based Diet*

"Considering *No Meat Athlete* is about eating a plant-based diet and running distances most people don't even like to drive, Matt Frazier presents the tools and information he shares in a way that is downright approachable, leaving his readers energized with a sense of possibility."

—**Brendan Brazier**, ultramarathon runner and author of *Thrive*

"Inspiring, encouraging, and packed with practical information, this is a book that will help anyone at any fitness level learn to eat and train for optimal plant-powered health."

—**Virginia Messina, M.P.H., R.D.**, author of *Vegan for Life* and *Vegan for Her*

"This book is a fantastic, no-fuss, no-judgment approach to plant-based eating and fitness. Whether you're curious, brand-new to this, or just keeping the blade sharp—get educated, get fed, get fit—read this book."

—**Osher Günsberg**, TV host, *Australian Idol*

". . . filled with practical advice, solid nutrition information, running tips, training plans, and recipes to fuel athletes of all abilities . . . a comprehensive guide to what you need to be healthy and fit while eating a whole-foods, plant-based diet."

—**Reed Mangels, Ph.D., R.D.**, co-author of *Simply Vegan* and *The Dietitian's Guide to Vegetarian Diets*

"If you were not feeling inspired or empowered before reading this book, you certainly will after. *No Meat Athlete* is the plant-based fuel that will keep you running strong!"

—**Terry Walters**, author of *Clean Food* and *Clean Start*

Foreword by **BRENDAN BRAZIER,** Ironman,
Ultramarathon Champion, and author of
the bestselling book *Thrive*

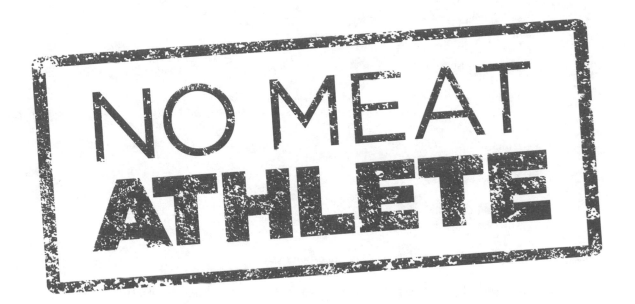

RUN ON PLANTS AND DISCOVER YOUR FITTEST, FASTEST, HAPPIEST SELF

MATT FRAZIER
Ultramarathoner and founder of NoMeatAthlete.com

with Matthew Ruscigno, M.P.H., R.D.

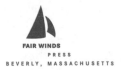

FAIR WINDS
PRESS
BEVERLY, MASSACHUSETTS

© 2013 Fair Winds Press
Text © 2013 Matt Frazier
Chapter 3 and recipes on pages 99, 101, and 147 © 2013 Matthew Ruscigno, M.P.H., R.D.

First published in the USA in 2013 by
Fair Winds Press, a member of
Quayside Publishing Group
100 Cummings Center
Suite 406-L
Beverly, MA 01915-6101
www.fairwindspress.com

All rights reserved. No part of this book may be reproduced or utilized, in any form or by any means, electronic or mechanical, without prior permission in writing from the publisher.

17 16 15 14 13   2 3 4 5

ISBN: 978-1-59233-578-7

Digital edition published in 2013
eISBN: 978-1-61058-909-3

Library of Congress Cataloging-in-Publication Data
Frazier, Matt.
 No meat athlete : run on plants and discover your fittest, fastest, happiest self / Matt Frazier with Matthew Ruscigno.
     pages cm
 Includes bibliographical references and index.
 ISBN 978-1-59233-578-7 (paperback)
 1. Runners (Sports)--Nutrition. 2. Athletes--Nutrition. 3. Physical fitness--Nutritional aspects. 4. Vegan cooking. 5. Veganism--Health aspects. 6. Running. I. Ruscigno, Matthew. II. Title.
 TX361.R86F72 2013
 641.5'636--dc23
                                2013024585

Cover design: Quayside Publishing Group
Cover photos: top left by Takao Suzuki; bottom left by Bren Dendy
Book design: Mighty Media
Book layout: Sporto

Printed and bound in the United States

The information in this book is for educational purposes only. It is not intended to replace the advice of a physician or medical practitioner. Please see your health care provider before beginning any new health program.

To Erin:

Your unwavering support through every change of course (just when things were starting to feel comfortable!) means the world to me.

Ten percent of author royalties from this book are donated to animal sanctuaries, including Farm Sanctuary, www.farmsanctuary.org. Thank you for your support in helping to end the mistreatment of animals.

CONTENTS

FOREWORD

Even as interest in plant-based diets grows and this healthy lifestyle becomes a more common part of mainstream culture, people are often still surprised to hear that such a diet, free of animal products, is more than adequate to fuel active lifestyles—from basic recreation for fitness to serious athletic endeavors.

They're even more shocked when I tell them, in my books and in talks throughout North America, that I chose this diet precisely because of what it could do for me as an athlete. When I made the decision in high school to try to become a professional endurance athlete, I experimented with all kinds of diets to find the one that would best support my dream. In the process of experimentation, I discovered that a plant-based diet stood alone as the one which most effectively allowed me to recover quickly from workouts, despite what coaches and others around me believed. The decreased recovery time between workouts that resulted from my new diet allowed me to train harder and more often than the competition, and ultimately, I see this advantage as the reason I succeeded in becoming a professional Ironman triathlete and have twice won the Canadian 50K ultramarathon championship.

The benefits of adopting a plant-based diet, though, go far beyond athletic performance. It's no secret that the standard American diet of processed and nutrient-devoid food has wreaked havoc on our health as a society, with obesity levels even among children soaring to all-time highs as a result. But what's not nearly as often talked about is that there exists a simple solution that can be implemented on the level of the individual—adopting a nutrient-rich, whole-food, plant-based diet. Almost immediately, such a diet can lead to lower levels of stress, better sleep, and a better mood. And longer-term, it has been shown to dramatically lower the incidence of heart disease and certain cancers, the leading killers in our society.

Environmentally speaking, eating plants over meat makes sense. Less land, water, and fossil fuel goes in the production of plants, and fewer CO_2 emissions are produced. It's simply a matter of efficiency; more nutrition (micronutrients) can be gained while spending less of each natural resource to get it.

And regardless of what you may believe about the right or wrong of raising animals for food, the way our current food system treats these animals—with its emphasis on factory farming and profit above all else—is hard to stomach.

It's incredible that a solution so simple as adopting a plant-based, whole-food focused diet can have such a large impact on all of the above areas. And yet, even when presented with the clear benefits of a plant-based diet, the vast majority of people still consider this lifestyle to be far more extreme than could ever work in their lives. And so they do little, and as a result, not much changes.

That's where *No Meat Athlete* comes in. If there's a single reason such a huge community of active, passionate people has sprouted up around *No Meat Athlete*—you've probably seen them in their running carrot shirts—it's this: Considering the website is about eating a plant-based diet and running distances most people don't even like to drive (a lifestyle many would consider "extreme"), Matt Frazier presents the tools and information he shares in a way that is downright approachable, leaving his readers energized with a sense of possibility and thinking, "Hey, I could actually do this." Matt's approach to health and fitness is informed, welcoming, and completely nonjudgmental, with a constant emphasis on simplicity and practicality (rather than absolute perfection) when it comes to diet and fitness choices.

The food and philosophy in the book you're holding represent a drastic improvement over the way most people—even many active and health-conscious people—fuel their daily lives. But the approach here isn't about being rigid or mechanical in your diet and exercise habits or making big sacrifices in your day-to-day life in return for incremental improvements at the highest levels of athletic performance.

Instead, it's about the bigger picture—that of making broad changes to your diet and exercise habits, changes that will have a lasting impact on your quality of life and the lives of those you share the planet with. It's about making this lifestyle work, even within the framework of the busy career and family lives most of us lead. And most importantly, it's about approaching these changes intelligently and deliberately, in a manner that's intended—above all else—to make sure that this time, they last.

Congratulations on deciding to make a difference. Get started now, and it won't be long before your body is thanking you.

—**Brendan Brazier,** best-selling author of *Thrive*

INTRODUCTION

As I passed the twenty-two-mile marker, I felt everything slipping away. I had been here before: the point in a race where you realize that your goal is too big, that today is not your day.

You hang on for a while longer, give it everything you've got for a few minutes, and wonder why the pace you've held for five or ten or twenty-two miles suddenly feels so hard. Then at some point, either because your body shuts down or you decide that failing will hurt less than your legs currently do, you give up. That's where I was. Hanging on, staving off the inevitable for just a few more minutes.

Maybe I had no business being here. As I looked around me and saw all these serious marathoners, athletes truly deserving of the label "runner," I felt like I didn't belong. I was a normal guy who somehow fell into running, not a runner.

My Journey to the Greatest Marathon in the World

Seven years prior, I ran my first marathon after two college buddies and I decided we'd do one, even though none of us knew much about running. But we were all in decent shape, so we aimed high.

And we didn't just set out to run a marathon. We were going to do better. We were going to run it fast enough to qualify for the Boston Marathon, the most famous and prestigious race in the world and one steeped in history as the world's oldest annual marathon. Every year, about 20,000 people run the race, with the support of half a million cheering, partying spectators on Patriots' Day, a state holiday known affectionately in Boston as "Marathon Monday."

The problem is, everyone wants to run Boston, but the course can only accommodate so many runners. To limit entrants and position the race as one meant for serious runners, the Boston Athletic Association imposed strict qualifying requirements in 1970. ("This is not a jogging race," stated the application to the 1970 marathon.) This restriction, of course, only added to the prestige of the race, igniting the desire of marathoners everywhere to earn the right to call themselves "Boston qualifiers." For us, as males under thirty-five years old, that meant running our marathon in 3 hours, 10 minutes, and 59 seconds or faster—a 7:17 minute per mile pace, for 26.2 miles.

We trained hard and put the miles in—at first. Then the aches, pains, midterms, and college parties happened.

Shockingly, all three of us made it to the start line of our marathon in San Diego. Training hadn't been great, but we'd done enough to believe we could finish. And somehow, though it was the most painful day any of us had ever experienced, we did just that.

Unfortunately, it took us a sobering four hours and fifty-three minutes—*a hundred minutes slower* than it would have taken to qualify for Boston. It was a reality check that we probably deserved, after thinking we were going to achieve (on our first try, no less) something that many serious, dedicated, seasoned marathoners never will.

My friends, like reasonable people, gave up on Boston. We had been proven wrong, fed the proverbial slice of humble pie. Today, they both keep in shape, but as far as I know, neither of them has plans to run another marathon. They've moved on.

I couldn't.

Seven years later, here I was. Just four miles—and half an hour—from doing it. From qualifying for Boston! So close and yet I was about to let everyone down—friends, family, and readers.

Yes, readers. I'm referring to the 500 or so people who had been following my training through my running and food blog, then just six months old. After my last marathon, I had begun to feel frustrated that with all the improvements I had made as a runner, I was still ten minutes shy of qualifying for Boston. Pushing myself too hard, I injured my knee a few weeks later, and (for what must have been the hundredth time) I wondered whether Boston just wasn't in the cards for me.

We trained hard and put the miles in—at first. Then the aches, pains, midterms, and college parties happened.

How I Came to Give a Plant-Based Diet a Try

That frustration and injury, it turns out, are what ultimately led me to become vegetarian. For a few years, I had felt a mild ethical pull to stop eating animals. But as an athlete, as someone whose identity was so intertwined with this quest to make it to Boston, I wouldn't let it happen.

Like most people, I was completely oblivious to the fact that there were world-class athletes, especially in endurance sports, who were out there competing with the best on 100 percent plant-based diets—no meat, no dairy, no eggs. And so, without knowing there were others out there doing it, I asked myself the same questions anyone else would have:

Where would I get protein? How could I possibly get enough calories to recover from 50 or 60 miles of running every week when I couldn't eat meat?

It was just too risky, I thought. I phased out red meat and pork and felt a little better about my food choices, but that was as far as I was willing to go.

Yet, as I started to plateau around the 3:20:00 mark (and especially after I got hurt), I began to have doubts about how far my current training and diet could take me. I had reached enough of a plateau that I no longer felt that if I just kept doing what I was doing, I'd get there. That approach had worked for a while, but not anymore. So the status quo wasn't as appealing as it had been before.

> *It felt almost unfair that I was able to work out as hard as I did and still recover in time for the next workout.*

I didn't want to do anything that would slow me down. Yet, as I started to learn about the health benefits of a high-plant diet (and some of the long-term health reasons for eschewing animal products, especially dairy), I wondered whether something like this could actually make me faster, if I was careful about how I did it.

And so I made the leap—sort of. I stopped eating my beloved chicken breasts and turkey burgers and cut most of the dairy out of my diet. I was left with fish as my only protein source, at least as I defined "protein source" back then.

Within just two weeks, I started to notice I didn't really need fish. I could get the protein I needed from beans, nuts, grains, and even green vegetables, and I felt just as full after a hearty (and surprisingly tasty) vegetarian meal as I did when I ate fish for dinner. I had become aware of elite vegan athletes like Brendan Brazier and was learning from them. And I felt better than ever, with more energy than I could remember having since I was a kid!

Gradually, I cut out the fish, and having never been an egg eater, I was left with occasionally eating cheese as the only animal product in my diet (something I eventually cut out entirely).

And all the while, I was rehabbing my knee injury, still thinking about Boston, and excitedly writing about my new diet on my blog.

A month or so after I started eating this way, I went on a run that I will never forget. It was my first attempt at a long run since the doctor had cleared me to resume running normally, and I didn't expect much. It was twelve miles, on a route that I ran regularly when I was healthy. This time, I was just hoping that nothing hurt.

To my surprise, I got home six minutes earlier than planned. That might not sound like a whole lot, but over twelve miles, six minutes is thirty seconds per mile. If I could improve my marathon pace by that much, that would be all I needed to get to Boston! And this after two months of next to zero running—could it be the diet?

From there, it felt like I was running downhill all summer. I ran my fastest half marathon, then my fastest 5K. I put in the strongest sixteen weeks of marathon training I've ever done, without injury, burnout, or fatigue from overtraining. Don't get me wrong, I worked hard—but it felt almost unfair that I was able to work out as hard as I did and still recover in time for the next workout.

All of this brought me to the moment I described at the beginning of this introduction—a windy day in October 2009, in Corning, New York, when I was twenty-two miles into the Wineglass Marathon with a half hour left until the race clock hit 3:11. I was within striking distance of the goal I had worked so hard for during the past seven years of my life. And I didn't think I was going to make it.

I had felt great for most of the race, despite a noticeable headwind and a course that wasn't quite as flat as I had expected. I had been able to run slightly faster than the required 7:17 pace to qualify for Boston, and for the first half of the race, I was sure I could do it.

Then miles fifteen, sixteen, and seventeen happened. If you've ever run a marathon, you probably know the feeling, where you start to notice that it takes just a little bit more work to move your legs. And you want to tell yourself, "I'm almost done," but you realize you've still got ten miles to go. You're not even close.

By mile twenty, I could feel it slipping away. Mile twenty-one was worse. As if it weren't enough to get this close only to fail again, I dreaded the thought of having to tell all the readers pulling for me that I had choked. All the work that had gone into this, down the drain. Not that it really would have been wasted, but of course you don't think of that when you're twenty miles into a marathon and facing the realization that you're not going to do the sole thing you've worked so hard to do. I envisioned a sad ride home and a miserable few weeks as I figured out what to do next. The idea of just abandoning the blog, never posting about the race (or ever again), flashed through my mind.

By the time I hit the twenty-two-mile marker, I had clocked two straight 7:30s, giving up almost 30 seconds from my goal pace. And there was no reason to think things would turn around. If anything, they'd just keep on getting worse, like they had at the end of every other marathon I'd run. I waited for the meltdown.

The meltdown, though, held off. And then an idea hit me.

If somehow, just somehow, I could do two more 7:30s, that would leave me with 2.2 miles to go at a 7:15 pace to sneak in under 3:10:59 and qualify.

Running a 7:15 right then and there would have seemed impossible in my current state. Why I had any faith that I could speed up during the last two miles of a marathon is beyond me; the final miles have always been the slowest in my previous races. But if I knew that I only had two miles left, that all the pain I'd gone through would be worth it if I could just leave it all on the course and really suffer for just fifteen minutes before collapsing in the grass, then maybe I could make it happen.

Surprisingly to me, the first part of my plan worked. Talking to myself, grimacing in pain, and doing what probably looked more like shuffling than running, I hung onto that 7:30 pace for miles twenty-three and twenty-four. At this point I was skipping water stops altogether, not even looking up at the volunteers' faces to say, "Thank you for helping." I was really, really hurting and about as focused as I've ever been.

When I started mile twenty-five, I said out loud to myself, "There's got to be more." I never talk to myself, and when I see people do it in movies, I gag and think that nobody really does that. But I did. I didn't mean "I know there's more, let's see it." Rather, I meant "If you're going to do this, then you have got to give more than you realize you have available to give."

I started speeding up, feeling sort of liberated in the realization that if this pace were too fast and I crashed during the last mile, then it wouldn't matter because I wouldn't have qualified anyway if I didn't go fast.

In other words, I had nothing to lose.

The twenty-fifth mile turned directly into the wind for a few hundred yards. Just when I thought I had survived and the course turned away from the wind, I found myself looking straight up a hill. But I didn't care about any of this. I just kept running hard, feeling almost reckless, and when I got to the mile marker, I looked at my watch and was overjoyed to see that it read 7:10.

Finally, the twenty-sixth mile—this was it. If I could do what I had just done, one more time, then I'd make it. Feeling this good caused me to speed up even more. I remember almost nothing of the last mile, except that I kept looking at my watch and being surprised that time was passing so quickly. A good thing, because I knew I was running fast enough. When I saw the twenty-six-mile marker and glanced at my watch, I knew I was home.

I sprinted the last 385 yards to the finish across a bridge, lined on one side with people. Among the chorus of voices, I heard someone yelling "Run fast!" and later found out it was my wife, Erin. I was going to qualify for Boston.

I raced the clock to cross the line in under 3:10:00 (remember, a 3:10:59 would have done it). I thought I lost that battle because my watch said 3:10:04 when I finished, but

I later found out that my chip time, the official one, was 3:09:59. I stumbled through the finish corral in a daze while someone put a medal on me and gave me a Mylar blanket.

The first person I saw was Erin, and she came and hugged me, screaming, "You did it Matt, you qualified for Boston!"

All I could say back was "I did it." As I said it, my eyes welled up, just as they had the dozens, maybe hundreds, of times I had envisioned this moment over the past seven years. I had earned a spot in the world's greatest marathon.

Was It the Plant-Based Diet?

I don't like to say that taking ten minutes off my previous best to qualify for Boston was entirely due to my new diet—there are just so many factors that can affect a given training cycle that I don't think it's fair to assume that any one was the reason. But there are two things I can say without question:

> ▶ I lost 5 pounds within the first two weeks of giving up most dairy and all meat, and I didn't lose any strength (as measured by how much weight I was lifting in the gym). That was a significant drop from my starting weight of 145, and over the course of ten or twenty miles, having to carry that much less weight makes a big difference.

> ▶ As I said previously, I was able to recover from workouts faster than at any other point in my life. I was putting in three extremely hard (for me) running workouts each week, with easy runs in between, along with some strength training. The fact that I dealt with no injury issues and was able to complete the assigned workouts (especially after just having come off an injury) was remarkable for me.

I believe it's these two factors that are responsible for the huge improvement I experienced, when prior to that I had begun to plateau. The weight loss was undoubtedly a result of my new diet—my weight had been steady before, and as soon as I changed my diet, I lost weight (thankfully, it stabilized at about seven pounds below my previous weight). The improved recovery is tougher because it's more subjective and could be the result of other factors. But what I've since learned, whenever I've had the chance to interview an elite plant-based athlete for my blog, is that they all cite the exact same benefit of the diet—decreased recovery time, with reduced incidence of injury as just one consequence.

Will Adopting a Plant-Based Diet Make You Stronger/ Faster/Fitter/Lighter?

I think so. And if you're curious enough to ask, it's worth giving it a try. I've thought a lot about what effect my vegetarian (and eventually vegan) diet has had in my life as a runner, and as one who is staunchly opposed to preaching about diet, I've tried to be as fair about it as I could possibly be.

After I qualified for Boston, feeling some confidence in my newfound resistance to injury, I got into ultramarathons, running two fifty-mile trail races within a few months of each other, along with several 50Ks that year. Most recently, I completed my first 100-mile race, an effort that saw me running for over 28 straight hours.

To me, that's saying something: at the very least, I can conclude that a plant-based diet hasn't hindered me like I used to be so convinced it would. What's more, there are elite vegan athletes in just about any sport you look at—endurance sports in particular, where Scott Jurek is one of the most dominant ultramarathoners to ever live and currently holds the American record of 165.7 miles in twenty-four hours, but also in speed and strength sports. Look at Mac Danzig, an elite mixed martial arts fighter. If you've ever seen this sport on television, I don't need to tell you that you've got to be in incredible physical condition to even survive a few minutes of a bout. Mac and many others maintain that kind of condition on diets free of animal products. Indeed, they choose a plant-based diet because it allows them to most effectively train and perform.

The benefits go beyond just short-term fitness and performance in sports, however. Many studies have linked animal protein to increased risk for heart disease and certain cancers, for example. And although you won't hear me preach about them much, there are many other, non-health-related benefits of a diet like this one. I've mentioned that the initial reason for my interest in vegetarianism was because I started to not feel right about eating animals—and what I've learned since then about factory farming and the way animals are (mis)treated in the process has only made that conviction stronger. There's also the enormous benefit to the environment of adopting a plant-based diet; some studies show that eating this way reduces one's carbon footprint even more than giving up your car!

How to Use This Book

I envision several types of people reading and benefiting from this book. There's the person who is already a vegetarian, already an athlete, but knows there's another level to both and wants to get there. There's the athlete who still eats meat but is what I call veg-curious. There are the vegetarians and vegans who want to get in shape and stop eating the junk food that, while technically vegan, isn't doing their body any favors. And of course, there's the newbie to both: the (currently) sedentary individual who doesn't eat particularly well and is ready to make some serious changes.

I've divided the book into two sections that can each stand on its own and be read in the order you choose. **Section I: Plant-Based Nutrition for Athletes**, is entirely about diet. It covers a philosophy of healthy eating that's simple and logical, without depending on calorie-counting or lots of confusing numbers. Starting from that foundation, we'll talk about the most effective way to transition to a plant-based diet, using the principles of habit change to make sure that it sticks. From there, we'll go into some of the nitty-gritty nutrition information. And after that, the focus of the remainder of the section is on planning and cooking meals (hint: you'll need to do this!) that are delicious and will get you the nutrients and calories you need as an athlete. Of course, there are plenty of healthy, filling, and delicious plant-based recipes for athletes at the end of the section, including recipes for fueling your workouts.

Running is the fastest way for ordinary people (like me, not super athletes) to do extraordinary things.

Section II: Running on Plants, outlines an approach to getting started as a runner, again using the principles of habit change to maximize your chances of success with it. From there, we'll get into more advanced training concepts, including a natural, plant-based strategy for fueling your workouts and recovery. And finally, I provide training programs for 5K, 10K, and half marathon distances.

Which brings me to a big question—why running, as opposed to other types of exercise? The biggest reason, as I see it, is that running is the fastest way for ordinary people (like me, not super athletes) to do extraordinary things. Most people consider running a marathon (remember, that's 26.2 miles) pretty extraordinary. What might surprise you, though, is that I believe *almost anyone can run a marathon if they're dedicated enough to put in the time and the miles.* You can't make a statement like that about, say, tennis or golf. These sports are fun and require exercise, but only a few people have the gifts to do something amazing with them, the way many people can with running (and other endurance sports). What's more, training for a race (whether it's a 5K, a half marathon, or even an ultramarathon) has the power to transform so many things about your life, not just your body. Your discipline, mental clarity, happiness, and your sense of structure and purpose in life—the list goes on.

With that, let's get started!

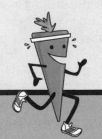

PLANT-BASED NUTRITION FOR ATHLETES

CHAPTER 1

FOOD AND NUTRITION PHILOSOPHY
(When Did Eating Become So Complicated?)

Visit any supermarket today and you'll see shelves lined with hundreds of items that just a few decades ago would have scarcely been recognized as food.

- ▶ Yogurt in a tube
- ▶ Lunchables
- ▶ Pasteurized processed cheese food
- ▶ Cheese in a CO_2 can
- ▶ Pepsi Cease Fire, designed—no joke—to put out the fire in your mouth caused by spicy Doritos Degree Burn

A lot of this—actually, all of it—is junk. Yet, what about all the "health food" we now have because of modern technology? Certainly, we're better off because of that, right? You don't even have to visit a specialty health store to find most of the following:

- ▶ Margarine fortified with omega-3 fatty acids
- ▶ Breads and milk pumped full of extra vitamins and minerals
- ▶ Soda that tastes sweet but has zero calories
- ▶ Multivitamins that provide us with ten times the amount of the vitamins and minerals we need each day
- ▶ Lab-designed meal replacement shakes for any diet you happen to be on

Much of the food people buy these days is so loaded with preservatives that it will never even rot! With all of this high-tech food available, it seems like we should be healthier than ever. You can walk into the health section of any bookstore and find hundreds of options promising to solve all your problems with the latest and greatest diet approach.

And yet rates of obesity in adults and children continue to grow, raising the risk of serious diseases, such as heart disease, stroke, diabetes, and certain cancers. It's said that our generation might be the first that fails to outlive its parents.

What Happened?

Food used to be simple. Tens of thousands of years ago, before the development of agriculture, our ancestors hunted and gathered. Nuts, legumes, roots, fruits, vegetables, meat when it was available, and little else. There were no artificial preservatives, and most ways of preserving food had not been discovered. We ate what we acquired quickly, before it could rot or be stolen by another human being or animal, because the next meal was rarely a sure thing. We didn't know what protein, fats, or carbohydrates were, much less antioxidants and free radicals.

But with all these seeming disadvantages compared to what we have at our disposal today, there was one huge factor our ancestors had going for them that we no longer have: *Back then, if a food tasted good, it was almost certainly good for you.* In fact, that's precisely why it tasted good. If you've never thought much about evolution, it's worth taking a second to understand how beautifully elegant the process is.

A Two-Minute Lesson in Evolution

According to the theory of evolution, our bodies evolved over millions of years to thrive on the foods and in the environmental conditions that existed at the time. Without getting into anything remotely technical, how does this work?

Let's think about it. A child with, say, a nut allergy, who lived in an area where nuts were one of the only available foods, didn't stand a good chance of surviving to adulthood. And so he could not pass his genes (and a predisposition to nut allergies) on to his own children. Another child, whose body thrived on nuts, however, would more likely grow up strong, father children who also liked nuts, and live happily ever after. (Until he is old and slow and eaten by a tiger whose body thrives on people.)

Over time (and I mean a *long* time), genes that did well with the available foods propagated throughout the tribe, while those that were incompatible with the available food were systematically removed from the gene pool, as their carriers died before they could pass those genes on.

It works the same with tastes. Why do fat and sugar taste so good? Because they're incredibly valuable sources of energy! Fat contains more than twice the calories (by weight) of other nutrients, and sugar can quickly be converted to usable energy. Back before your next meal was such a sure thing, if you had the rare opportunity to consume a large amount of either fat or sugar, you'd have been crazy not to take it.

And so natural selection rewarded those who loved the taste of fat and sugar. People who sought out these valuable nutrients had an advantage over those who enjoyed the taste of, say, nutrient-poor tree bark, and were more likely to live long enough to procreate. And so in this manner, the genes for craving fat and sugar were passed down for thousands of generations.

You see, there's nothing inherently bad about fat and sugar. But here's the catch: for the millions of years during which most of our evolution has occurred, fat and sugar were scarce. Fast-forward to the present day, and acquiring fat and sugar is as easy as swinging by 7-Eleven. While a buffalo kill might have been a rare treat back in the day, you can now get a Big Mac and a Coke from a McDonald's drive-through for five bucks. What's more, it used to be just about impossible to eat too much fat and sugar: they were only available as parts of whole foods, not extracted and concentrated as they are today. (There was certainly no way to extract high-fructose corn syrup from corn.)

For the millions of years during which most of our evolution has occurred, fat and sugar were scarce. Fast-forward to the present day and acquiring fat and sugar is as easy as swinging by 7-Eleven.

Taking in 30 grams of fat meant eating a large piece of meat or a whole bunch of nuts, which filled up your stomach to the point that it signaled to your brain "Enough, stop eating!" But nowadays, you can get almost that much fat in 2 tablespoons (28 ml) of oil, which takes up little room in your stomach and does nothing to trigger a "that's enough-stop-stuffing-your-face" response.

The same goes for sugar. When we eat more sugar than we can use right away, most of it gets stored as fat. This wasn't a big problem when the only way to get sugar was to eat whole fruit—there's only so much fruit you can eat before you're full. But now we can simply drink sugar-rich juice, skipping the fiber that serves to fill us up. (Remember, we evolved in the presence of whole foods, so every edible part of the food serves our bodies in ways scientists still don't fully understand.)

In the worst case, we now consume sugar in ultra-concentrated syrups, such as those found in most sodas and almost any packaged dessert, and in our breakfast cereal, bread, muffins, bagels, salad dressings, ketchup, barbecue sauce, pasta sauce, applesauce, yogurt, soup, pretzels, chicken strips, and sports drinks—oh yeah, and in our medicine. And we wonder why we're getting fat.

What Else Is Wrong?

Highly processed oils, refined sugars, and dairy products (more on this later) are what I believe to be the biggest culprits in the terribly unhealthy standard American diet. But that's not to say they're the only problems.

This book is about solutions, not problems, so I'll mention these other issues only briefly here to give some rationale for the recommendations that follow throughout the first half of this book.

1. OVER-PROCESSING

We've already talked about processing as it pertains to extracted oils and added refined and concentrated sugars, but the problem is a lot more pervasive than that. Grains are one of the most common refined foods. Wheat, for example, is usually stripped of the fibrous, nutrient-rich bran before being ground into the pure white flour that makes so many of our breads, bagels, and pastas—similar to white rice, which is brown before processing. The removed fiber and nutrients are what are supposed to fill us up to regulate how much we can eat. Without them, though, we get no such stop sign.

Many "foods" are nothing but assemblies of many not-quite-foods that have been processed and combined with artificial ingredients. Look at the ingredients in most popular snack foods or sodas. There's nothing there that's even close to a whole food!

And it's not just traditional factories that churn out foods with the nutrients removed. Often, it happens before our fruits and vegetables even leave the farm.

2. LOW-NUTRIENT PRODUCE

It used to be that if you wanted a tomato in the winter, you were out of luck. Not anymore! Now, you can get just about any food, just about any time. Food is shipped in from all over the world, often from a farm dedicated to producing that single food and nothing else.

Do the tomatoes you get in the winter taste like those you get from your local farmers market in the summer? Of course not. The ones trucked in over the winter are usually pink, not red, and they're as devoid of flavor as they are color. And you know what that means they're also devoid of? Nutrition. From the time a food is picked to the time it arrives on your plate, several weeks often pass. For the food to be ripe when you eat it, farmers need to pick that fruit before it's ready to be picked, which means it hasn't had the time to develop the nutrition (or flavor) that it would if it were to be consumed shortly after picking.

What's more, much factory farming happens in a way that, over time, depletes the nutrients in the soil. Although sustainable farming practices ensure that crops are rotated year-to-year and grown in a manner and quantity that won't deplete the soil over time, much of what we see in grocery stores is not grown that way. The result is that with each and every passing season, the fruits and vegetables we consume are becoming less nutritious and mineral-rich. A 2004 study, published in the *Journal of the American College of Nutrition*, examined the nutrient content of forty-three food crops and found that levels of six nutrients and minerals, including protein, iron, calcium, and potassium, had significantly declined between 1950 and 1999, concluding that tradeoffs between yield and nutrient content may be to blame.

3. REDUCTIONIST FIXES TO NUTRITION PROBLEMS AREN'T ALWAYS THE SOLUTION

At the heart of many of the problems with our food today is the idea that nutrients are nutrients and vitamins are vitamins, and it doesn't matter in what context we get them as long as we get them somehow. If we need more vitamin E in our diet, just add it to the milk! If it's iron you seek, put it in the bread! Don't want to eat any food that's vitamin-rich? Just take a multivitamin.

It's only recently that we're coming to understand how remarkably complex food—and the way our bodies handle it—is. As stated previously, humans evolved to eat the foods in our environment—the *whole* foods, not simply the juice or the syrup or the oil of those foods.

We depend on the precise, not-fully-understood interactions between our bodies and *all* the components that make up a food. We can't simply take the omega-3s from one food, put them in another, and expect our bodies to accept that. This fallacy of scientific reductionism, first pointed out to me by Michael Pollan in his manifesto *In Defense of Food*, explains why with so much supposed "health food" out there, as a society we're only getting more unhealthy. As Pollan wrote in 2007 in the *New York Times*:

> . . . people don't eat nutrients, they eat foods, and foods can behave very differently than the nutrients they contain. Researchers have long believed . . . that a diet high in fruits and vegetables confers some protection against cancer. So naturally they ask, "What nutrients in those plant foods are responsible for that effect?" One hypothesis is that the antioxidants in fresh produce—compounds like beta carotene, lycopene, vitamin E, etc.—are the X factor. It makes good sense: these molecules . . . vanquish the free radicals in our bodies, which can damage DNA and initiate cancers. At least that's how it seems to work in the test tube. Yet as soon as you remove these useful molecules from the context of the whole foods they're found in, as we've done in creating antioxidant supplements, they don't work at all. Indeed, in the case of beta carotene ingested as a supplement, scientists have discovered that it actually increases the risk of certain cancers. Big oops.

4. ENVIRONMENTAL AND ECONOMIC CONCERNS

It's no secret that much of the world lives in a manner that, with regard to our planet and natural resources, is unsustainable. When most people think of environmental problems, they picture smoke-belching factories obscuring the sky, toxic chemicals being dumped into streams, and gas-guzzling SUVs packed onto highways during rush hour.

What this picture of environmental destruction is missing, however, is the effect of our food choices. In reality, factory farming, particularly livestock production, is among the leading causes of our environmental woes, producing more greenhouse gases, for example, than all forms of transportation combined! Consider these facts about the effect on the environment of livestock alone, taken from *Livestock's Long Shadow*, a report from the Food and Agriculture Organization of the United Nations in 2006, which determined that the livestock industry is one of the two or three most significant causes of serious environmental problems, on local and global scales and all scales in between (the term livestock, as used here, comprises all farmed animals, including pigs, birds raised for their meat and eggs, and dairy cows):

- ▶ The expansion of livestock production is a major contributor to deforestation. For example, 70 percent of Latin American land that used to be Amazon forest is now pasture for livestock, and much of the other 30 percent is used for crops to feed this livestock.

- ▶ The livestock sector produces 18 percent of greenhouse gas emissions, more than the entire transportation sector.

- ▶ In the United States, livestock account for 55 percent of erosion and sediment, 37 percent of pesticide use, and half of antibiotic use.

- ▶ Thirty percent of the earth's land surface, which was once habitat for wildlife, is now used for livestock production—this is just one factor that leads the study's authors to suggest "the livestock sector may well be the leading player in the reduction of biodiversity."

It's pretty clear what a tremendous mess we human beings have gotten ourselves and our planet into. Without even touching ethical issues regarding the decision to eat animals, we've identified major problem areas—namely, our health and that of our environment, whose poor condition is largely the result of our food choices.

If we agree on the problems our current food situation has caused, let's now turn our attention to what we can do about it.

What's the Solution?

Yes, fortunately, there is one. The answer to our diet problems is remarkably simple, and it's the common thread that explains why so many wildly different diets work.

Let's take a look at a few popular diets to see whether you can identify what that common element is. (Note: When I use the word "diet" throughout this book, I usually mean "a way of eating," as opposed to the state of being on a diet, in which one temporarily cuts calories or radically changes what he or she eats, usually to quickly lose weight and gain it all back when the diet ends.)

The Paleo Diet

The Paleo diet is based on the same evolutionary arguments we've talked about here. The apparent goal of the Paleo diet is to replicate what we ate during most of our evolution, but given that certain Paleo foods are extinct or significantly different than they were during most of our evolutionary history, some sacrifices have to be made. (For example, selective agriculture has made many of the fruits we eat now much juicier and less fibrous than they were previously.)

Paleo focuses on high-protein and low-carbohydrate foods. Approved foods include meat from wild animals, fruits, vegetables, nuts, and tubers. No grains or dairy are allowed because those came about relatively late in our existence.

And it works for athletes, at least in the short run, as evidenced by the popularity of Paleo among competitive athletes, most notably the CrossFit crowd.

It's pretty clear what a tremendous mess we human beings have gotten ourselves and our planet into.

The Raw and Fruitarian Diets

Then there's raw foodism. Here, the idea is that cooking our food is a recent enough technological advance that our bodies haven't yet had a chance to adapt to the change. Therefore, our bodies are designed to eat foods in their natural, raw state. Certain enzymes that help with digestion, along with other nutrients, are denatured during the cooking process, rendering them ineffective at their jobs. Some raw foodists include raw dairy and meat products in their diet.

Raw's cousin, fruitarianism (similar to the 30 Bananas a Day or 80/10/10 diets, which center on eating primarily simple carbohydrates and low amounts of protein and fat), focuses more on fruit than vegetables. The diet is composed of about 80 percent carbohydrates, includes no animal products whatsoever, and is entirely raw in its purest form. And Michael Arnstein, the most visible leader of the movement, has won the Vermont 100-miler and placed highly in the Leadville 100, one of the most famous ultramarathons in the world.

The Vegan Diet

And of course, there's veganism, which I usually call "plant-based," because this book is about eating for health more than it is about ethics. But even within the realm of veganism, there are differing versions.

Ultramarathon great Scott Jurek eats a traditionally balanced vegan diet (even if he consumes many more calories than the average vegan to fuel his 100-plus mile races). Then there's Brendan Brazier, *Thrive* author and former pro Ironman triathlete, who also eats plant-based foods, but focuses more on raw foods. The diets of both of these athletes include a relatively large amount of calories from fat, probably in the range of 25 percent.

But there's another version of the vegan diet that has gained a ton of traction, thanks largely to the 2011 runaway hit documentary *Forks Over Knives*. The documentary is based on the work of T. Colin Campbell, Ph.D., author of *The China Study*, and Caldwell Esselstyn, M.D., which links consumption of meat and dairy products to cancer and heart disease and advocates a "plant-based, whole foods diet". The diet is exactly what it sounds like—no animal products and no processed foods. Campbell and Esselstyn do not consider oils to be whole foods, for example, because in nature they only exist as parts of other foods, and so they advocate cooking with vegetable broth instead of even the olive oil that so many of us have considered healthy for so long.

The Common Thread

Clearly, the diets we've looked at are strikingly different on the surface, especially when you consider the wide variation in the ratios of protein, carbohydrate, and fat to which the different diets adhere. But have you noticed the fundamental element that they all share?

What they have in common is that each one of them focuses on whole foods, while avoiding processed foods and dairy. If you took those few steps and made no other changes to your current diet, you'd almost certainly experience major improvements in your health, as long as your food sources are varied to ensure you get a good mix of vitamins and nutrients.

Yes, making your diet healthy is really that simple.

How Should We Define "Whole Foods"?

I have yet to see a perfect definition of a "whole food." The problem is that for any food to go from its source (e.g., the ground, a tree, a stalk) to our plates requires some amount of processing, if you define the term loosely enough (e.g., sautéing or baking is a form of processing). And so most definitions rely on phrases like "processed as little as possible," which, of course, then leads to all kinds of questions as to what is meant by "as little as possible."

Let's not get hung up on the precise dividing line between whole foods and processed foods—there is no such line that everyone agrees on. Instead, the degree of processing is a continuum; the question should be, "How processed is it?" not "Is it processed?" Another important consideration is how much the food changes as it is processed. This is not the same consideration of how the food looks when it reaches our plates—tofu, for example, looks nothing like the soybeans from which it comes, but much of the integrity of the soybean remains in tofu. (Let's put aside the question of whether soy is healthy for now—we'll talk about that in chapter 3.)

Although I can't give you a precise test for distinguishing whole from processed foods, most foods are so far to one end of the spectrum or the other that you can fairly easily classify them as belonging to one group or the other (there are a few close calls, but not all that many). For instance:

- ▶ Baked potatoes? Sure, they're a whole food. Potato chips? No.
- ▶ A smoothie made from blended, whole fruits is still whole; fruit juice that a machine separates from the pulp isn't.
- ▶ Corn kernels cut away from the cob are still whole, corn syrup is not.
- ▶ And yes, meat is a whole food. Slim Jims are not.

What about Dairy?

We humans love our cows' milk. We're taught that it makes us strong and that all the calcium is good for our bones. But milk is not a health food. Remember when we talked about evolution, and how we evolved to thrive on the foods that were present in our environment? By that argument, I've got to admit that I don't think meat in small quantities—say, as a side dish for a few meals a week—is inherently unhealthy. (I'll talk about my reasons for choosing not to eat meat later in the chapter.) Dairy, though, is another story altogether.

Female mammals evolved to produce the perfect food for supporting a newborn for his or her first year of life—we know it as milk, of course. If a woman carried a gene (technically, several genes) for producing good milk, it increased the chances that her children (who would likely carry that same gene) were well-fed, lived through adulthood, and reproduced to pass on the gene. And so, just like we talked about before, over millions of years, milk gradually became the perfect food for infants.

Infants. Infants, I should point out, *of the same species.*

Humans didn't often drink cows' milk for most our evolution; it only came about with the development of agriculture 8,000 years or so ago. It seems unlikely that in a relatively short time period, humans could have evolved to thrive on, much less need,

We continue to drink cows' milk through adulthood and for our entire lives, making us the only species to drink milk beyond infancy.

cows' milk. What's more, we continue to drink cows' milk through adulthood and for our entire lives, making us the only species to drink milk beyond infancy.

Nature designed human milk for baby humans and cows' milk for baby cows. Cows' milk is formulated by nature to help an infant cow gain a thousand pounds in its first year. Should we be surprised, then, that when humans consume dairy, it's linked to certain reproductive cancers? Consider, for example, a 2001 Harvard Physician's Health Study that examined more than 20,000 U.S. male physicians and determined that those who consumed more than 2.5 servings of dairy products each day had a 34 percent higher risk of prostate cancer than those who consumed less than half a serving of dairy each day. Or a 2004 study published in the *American Journal of Clinical Nutrition* that found that women who drank more than one glass of milk per day (regardless of fat content) had double the ovarian cancer risk of those who drank one glass or less each day.

Many of us, Americans especially, grew up with the idea that cows' milk is the perfect food for humans, thanks largely to wildly successful advertising campaigns by the dairy industry. Who doesn't remember the milk mustache ads? Or the "Milk—It does a body good" slogan? In reality, it may do just the opposite.

So, Why Plant-Based?

First, let's get clear about the language. Throughout this book, you'll see me refer to this diet as "plant-based." What exactly does it mean?

To some, a "plant-based diet" means a vegan diet—no animal products, not even honey. To others, it simply means a diet that's "based" on plants, as in, you can eat a little cheese now and then or even a hamburger once in a while, as long as the vast majority of what you eat is plants.

Is a plant-based diet healthier than an omnivorous one? That's a tough one.

You could choose either definition and still benefit tremendously from the information and recipes in this book. *No Meat Athlete* is about health, not ethics, and it's my opinion that, all else being equal, two people eating plant-based diets using the two different definitions above won't notice dramatic differences when they compare their health to one another's. Thus, when I say "plant-based," I'm intentionally being vague. If you want it to mean strict veganism, that's great. If you want it to mean vegan, but you'll still eat ice cream once a month and put real butter on your popcorn, that works, too. Ethically, there's an enormous difference; I don't deny that, and I'm proud to call myself a true vegan. But in terms of your health, the two diets are nearly identical.

Is a plant-based diet healthier than an omnivorous one? That's a tough one. I believe I'm a lot healthier now that I'm vegan. It forces me to avoid fast food and countless other convenient but unhealthy foods that I used to eat. In my mind, there's no question that a well-planned, plant-based diet is healthier than the standard (terrible) American diet.

But how about compared to a whole-foods diet that happens to include a small amount of meat, eggs, and just a bit of dairy?

To me, it's not clear that one diet is necessarily healthier than the other. I'm fine to call it a tie. I just know that passing up a McDonald's is way easier for me now than it was before I was vegan, and as a result, I make so much more of my own food than I used to and eat so many more fruits and vegetables than before. For that aspect, I love it.

CHANGING YOUR LIFE, ONE MEAL AND ONE RUN AT A TIME

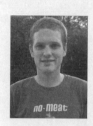

By Pete DeCapite

I've always been skinny. No matter what I ate, I could never put on many pounds. I went through a period in high school when I was so self-conscious about my weight that I ate everything that was high-fat. It was my goal to eat the opposite of healthy foods in hopes of gaining weight and looking more "normal." My usual day was filled with fast food and as many piles of meat as possible. Eventually, it worked, and during college I gained about thirty pounds. That might not sound like much, but added to a 130-pound frame, it felt like a ton.

That thirty pounds made me feel better about my appearance, but it took a toll on my health. I started feeling chest pains when I was only twenty years old, severe enough to make me lose my breath and kneel on the ground on multiple occasions. Finally, I went to a doctor and learned that my total cholesterol was around 250 and my triglycerides had reached 300. The numbers only substantiated how terrible I felt.

You would think this news would change my life overnight, that I would get serious about my health, and my diet would improve. But neither happened. I slipped back into my same routine of poor eating and little exercise. I was young, what harm could it do?

Then, in 2009 I got an email from my friend Matt Frazier, saying he was starting a blog called *No Meat Athlete*. It had a funny name and concept, so I read the first post. I wasn't into the whole vegetarian thing, but I tried a few recipes from his blog. After eating each meal, I felt better and more energetic. I didn't have the post-meal bloating and fatigue I was used to. One meal at a time, I went from a meat-and-potatoes guy to a vegetarian.

It took me almost a year to admit publically that I was a vegetarian, but at that point, I didn't care. I felt great, so why should I feel ashamed that I didn't need to eat meat with dinner to call it a meal? Over the next year, I continued on this path, and I eventually gave up dairy.

I started running, too. I signed up for the local 5K that I had run when I was a kid. The first couple of months were rough trying to get my stamina back, but with each run I grew stronger. My brother convinced me to go even farther and run a ten-miler, which I reluctantly did.

After each race, I always said that was it, that I had reached my goal, and now I would scale back and enjoy easier running. However, after my ten-miler I decided to do a half marathon. And soon after that, I signed up for a marathon, something I had told Matt would never happen.

In November 2011, I ran the Marine Corps Marathon, beating my goal of four hours by fourteen seconds. I then started running trails and ran my first ultramarathon, a 50K in Elkton, Maryland, two months later. The feelings of accomplishment were amazing. It is difficult to describe to a non-runner why I run, but once you hit that runner's high after hours of running, you just know.

Now I weigh around 140 pounds, and my cholesterol is under 200 and drops every time I get it checked. I feel like a completely different person than that guy who read that first *No Meat Athlete* email and thought his friend was a little crazy. My life truly changed, one meal and one run at a time.

Four Compelling Reasons to Choose a Plant-Based Diet

The rather equivocal viewpoints I've expressed in this chapter might have come as a surprise—aren't vegans supposed to defend their diet choices more adamantly than this?

Yes, many of us do, often with good reason. But if I can't honestly say with 100 percent certainty that a plant-based diet is healthier than a whole-foods–based omnivorous one, or that it offers a decided advantage for sports, I'm not going to make those claims.

But here's the thing—I don't need to. Even without taking a side in the debate about which is better, there are so many ways a plant-based diet makes me fitter, faster, and happier. Following are my reasons for choosing to eat a vegan diet.

1. Ethical considerations

The single most important factor behind my decision to be vegan is the fact that I cannot feel at peace about supporting the way tens of *billions* (not a typo, and not an exaggeration either) of thinking, feeling animals are treated each year on their way from birth to our plates.

Although I won't go further about ethical issues here, in the resources section at the end of this book you'll find a few films, websites, and books worth checking out if you'd like to learn more about how food animals are treated. (For many vegetarians, improving the way animals are treated becomes their biggest source of inspiration to make their diet change last.)

2. Recent science linking plant-based diets to long-term disease prevention

We hear so much about which diets are healthy and which are not. What are we supposed to believe?

And then how much research is enough? How do we then make recommendations? It's one thing to learn about nutritional sciences and another to formulate recommendations for groups of people.

Fortunately, vegetarians as a group have been studied for decades. In fact, it's no stretch to argue that more research has been done on the vegetarian diet than any other specific eating pattern in the United States, and it's long been noted in scientific studies that vegetarians tend to live longer and experience a lower incidence of disease than the general population. Can we say then, that a plant-based diet is the key to health? Unfortunately, it's not quite so simple.

In addition to eating more fruits and vegetables than the general population, vegetarians also eat fewer foods containing saturated fat and cholesterol, and they tend to smoke less and exercise more. But (and there's always a "but"), we've learned that all of these other factors, *on their own and apart from vegetarianism* are beneficial in reducing chronic disease and increasing longevity.

Is it vegetarianism, or simply the tendencies of vegetarians to partake in other healthy behaviors, that accounts for the lower incidence of disease and longer lifespans correlated with vegetarian diets?

Is it vegetarianism, or simply the tendencies of vegetarians to partake in other healthy behaviors, that accounts for the lower incidence of disease and longer lifespans correlated with vegetarian diets? Researchers, the smart bunch they are, had the same question. In particular, researchers affiliated with Seventh-Day Adventist universities found themselves in a unique position to study this issue. You see, they knew that most followers of the Seventh-Day Adventist Church don't smoke, they exercise regularly, and eat lots of fruits and vegetables. And about half of them, in the United States, are vegetarian. See where this is going?

These researchers created the Adventist Health Study, which followed 34,000 Adventists and recorded their habits, asking questions about how often they exercised, which vegetables they ate and how often, and which diseases they developed.

Much of the evidence about the benefits of vegetarianism comes from this group. Hundreds of subsequent studies have been done using the information gathered from these 34,000 people, who are nearly identical in habits, except that some of them eat meat and others do not (only a small percentage of this group is vegan). Researchers are now hard at work looking at a second Adventist Health Study, this time with a cohort of 125,000 people! Further, the percentage of Adventists eating a completely vegan diet has increased significantly since the time when the first study was done; this development allows researchers to draw conclusions not just about the effect a meat-free diet has on health, but also of a diet completely free of all animal products.

At the time this book was published, only a few research articles based on the study have come out in peer-reviewed journals. These preliminary results, as presented by lead researcher Gary Fraser, M.D., Ph.D., include the following:

> ► A *Diabetes Care* study published in 2009 showed that risk for type 2 diabetes and obesity was greatest among non-vegetarians and lowest for vegans. Risk increased incrementally based on how often animal products were consumed. This remained true even after factors like physical activity and body-mass index (BMI) were controlled for.

> ► A 2012 study concluded that vegan diets confer the lowest risk for overall cancer compared to other dietary patterns. Lacto-ovo vegetarian diets, which include dairy and eggs, but not flesh, were also found to be protective, but vegans, again, had the lowest risk for cancer compared with vegetarians and non-vegetarians.

> ► Finally, a definitive statement on vegetarianism comes from The Academy of Nutrition and Dietetics (formerly the American Dietetic Association), the world's largest organization of food and nutrition professionals. Although we've looked at just a few studies here, members of this organization consider all major nutrition studies, and hence provide an informed perspective. The statement from 2009 is worth quoting at length, considering the academy is *not* widely considered to be a pro-vegetarian group:

It is the position of . . . the Academy of Nutrition and Dietetics that appropriately planned vegetarian diets, including total vegetarian or vegan diets, are healthful, nutritionally adequate, and may provide health benefits in the prevention and treatment of certain diseases. Well-planned vegetarian diets are appropriate for individuals during all stages of the life cycle, including pregnancy, lactation, infancy, childhood, and adolescence, and for athletes. . . The results of an evidence-based review showed that a vegetarian diet is associated with a lower risk of death from ischemic heart disease. Vegetarians also appear to have lower low-density lipoprotein cholesterol levels, lower blood pressure, and lower rates of hypertension and type 2 diabetes than non-vegetarians. Furthermore, vegetarians tend to have a lower body mass index and lower overall cancer rates. Features of a vegetarian diet that may reduce risk of chronic disease include lower intakes of saturated fat and cholesterol and higher intakes of fruits, vegetables, whole grains, nuts, soy products, fiber, and phytochemicals.

3. Food variety

Another by-product that I didn't expect of going vegetarian was that within the first few months of doing so, I was eating dozens of foods that I had never tried before.

The average American probably doesn't eat more than a few dozen foods each year (ignoring, for the sake of argument, nutritionally worthless varieties of junk food). It's so easy to fall into a rut of grilling chicken breast, accompanying it with a starch like potatoes, rice, or pasta, and maybe throwing in a vegetable as an afterthought. I know because I ate this way for many years, thinking I ate about as healthily as one could.

But when you go plant-based, you need to get outside of your box and explore. Sure, there's no rule that says omnivores can't eat foods such as quinoa, kubocha squash, kale, rainbow chard, celeriac, and millet—but how many of them actually do?

Another by-product that I didn't expect of going vegetarian was that within the first few months of doing so, I was eating dozens of foods that I had never tried before.

4. Environmental benefits

In light of the statistics on the environmental effect of livestock production presented earlier in the chapter, it's easy to see how a plant-based diet can do more for the environment than almost any other individual choice. Aside from the vote with your dollar that you cast when you choose not to participate in that industry, the decision to go vegan reduces your indirect consumption of water and energy as well.

- On average, a person who doesn't eat meat or dairy indirectly consumes nearly 600 gallons of water per day *less* than a person who eats the average American diet, according to *National Geographic*.

- The amount of energy required from fossil fuel to produce 1 calorie of animal protein for human consumption is 25.4 calories, according to Cornell University Science News. To produce an equivalent amount of plant protein, it takes less than one-tenth that amount, 2.2 calories.

It's tough to argue that the environment (and those of us who live in it) wouldn't be a whole lot better off if more people chose a vegan diet. But even if you don't go all the way vegan—say, you go vegetarian or pescetarian (vegetarian or vegan, plus fish), or have a few meatless days each week, you'll still dramatically reduce your environmental footprint versus when you eat a traditional Western diet.

If you've made it this far, it's a safe bet you're on board. The fact that you picked up this book made you a pretty good candidate! Let's get on to the good stuff. In the next chapter, I'll present a guide to getting started, so you can jump right in before we get into the nitty-gritty details of a healthy plant-based diet for active people.

CHAPTER 2

GETTING STARTED: CREATING A HEALTHY, PLANT-BASED EATING HABIT

What I want you to do, before you do anything else, is start. This probably sounds obvious—what else is there to do first, right?

But so many of us, once inspired to make a big change in our lives, never bother to start. Instead, we go into planning mode: we want to make a meal plan, learn all the principles of the new diet, wait until all our bad food runs out, wait until next week—you get the point.

Planning is important, eventually. But for most people, it too easily becomes a form of procrastination. Then soon enough, life throws something else at you, you deal with it, and you never come back to starting.

Why Starting Small Is Crucial

Healthy habits aren't the result of willpower. They happen because when we take an action enough times—preceded by a consistent trigger and followed by some sense of reward—our brains build pathways that make the habit our natural response whenever that trigger occurs. Let's look at a few examples of how this "habit loop" looks when it comes to food.

For many people, there's no stronger instance of the trigger-action-reward loop than their morning cup of Joe. You wake up, roll out of bed, and feel groggy (trigger), then you make and drink your coffee or get it on the way to work (action), and the loop is completed when the aroma, flavor, warmth, and caffeine cause you to feel awake, alert, and happy (reward). The habit loop doesn't get much more textbook than that!

Look at the times throughout the day when we eat because of a stressful situation. We come home from work after a busy day, for example, and most of us go right for the fridge. This isn't necessarily a bad thing, especially if the food we're eating is healthy, but it serves to illustrate the power of the loop. The act of coming home from work is the trigger, the action is the eating, and the reward is that you relax as your stomach fills and you taste food that you enjoy. It's interesting to note that even after a particularly easy day at work, when our stress level isn't so high, we'll likely still fall into the pattern, simply because the act of walking in the door triggers us to perform the action of eating.

Of all the ways you can improve your odds of success, there's one that stands out as the most important: start small.

Just like your chest muscles get tired (and need a few days to recover) when you do bench presses at the gym, your willpower runs out when it's overworked by a difficult task.

Many studies show that willpower is like a muscle—it gets stronger or weaker depending on how much we exercise it, but more importantly, it fatigues. Just like your chest muscles get tired (and need a few days to recover) when you do bench presses at the gym, your willpower runs out when it's overworked by a difficult task.

Yet when most of us try to form a new habit—say, a new diet or fitness program—we try to attack it with willpower alone. If we're hoping to start going to the gym regularly, for example, we jump right into an hour-long workout. It feels great at first, when our willpower is still going strong. The next day, it's not quite as much fun, but still bearable. By the end of that week or the next, though, it often becomes a chore to get out the door as the TV, couch, and bag of chips start calling our name.

What happens in situations like this is that our willpower runs out before our brain can build a neural pathway to make going to the gym a habit.

Fortunately, research suggests that there are things we can do to engineer our habits to maximize our chances of success, such as always taking the desired action after a precise daily trigger. For example, if your goal is to eat a salad each day, you might choose to eat it after your daily three o'clock work appointment. Even more important, though, is that you make the habit *easy to stick with at first*.

CHOOSE WHOLE FOODS
FOR HIGH PERFORMANCE:
How an Ultrarunning Mother Gets It Done

By Meredith Murphy
Ultrarunner and acupuncturist, two-time finisher of the
Badwater Ultramarathon in California, a 135-mile footrace
from Death Valley to Mount Whitney

Before my daughter was born in 2009, I never had a hard time training and always got the miles and long runs in, but that all changed when she arrived. Now it is all about finding balance. I learned to love the jogging stroller, wake up before everyone else to run, and quietly run on the treadmill or do the stair stepper during nap time. I've also cut back my racing since she was born, and in her earlier years, had to find races where I could nurse her or pump breast milk. That surely throws a whole new aspect into race prep! I did a lot of races that were on looped courses, so it was easy to nurse her throughout.

As far as being vegetarian (pretty much vegan) and training, I do not use fancy gels or drinks or bars while training and racing, but rely on whole foods. I like granola bars, raw food bars, nuts, fruit, fruit juices, soy or almond milks, and peanut butter and jelly sandwiches. I have run the Badwater Ultramarathon twice, and eating a plant-based diet was quite a challenge because there is really not much in Death Valley in the way of vegetarian or vegan food. We bring all our food for almost a week: burritos, veggie burgers, baked tofu, hummus, pitas, tortillas, veggies and dip, and snack foods. During the race I ate a lot of fruit. It was my favorite thing to eat and the easiest on my stomach.

No matter the distance you are training for, what is important is eating high quality whole foods during training and all the time. When it is hard to carry things like fruit with me during a race, I look for high quality bars that are easy to fit in a pocket. I found, in my experience, that when I used fancy training and racing specific products, my stomach suffered. It took a long time, and a lot of money, to realize that my body just wanted real food!

Why? As I said previously, it takes time and many repetitions for your brain to build the pathway that eventually becomes a habit. In the case of eating a salad each afternoon, the trick is to make eating that salad enjoyable, so that you don't deplete your willpower each day that you eat it. If you don't love salad yet, do whatever it takes to make the salad delicious while you develop the habit. You'll want to eventually transition to healthier salads, but at first, establishing the habit loop is your only concern.

It takes time and many repetitions for your brain to build the pathway that eventually becomes a habit.

How do you do that? All sorts of ways. For example, use a dressing that's really tasty when you're getting started, even if it's not the healthiest in the world. Toss some croutons or candied nuts on top, or anything else that tastes good and varies the texture, if that'll help you get the ball rolling. Make it so you actually look forward to your salad—the complete opposite of having to burn up your willpower to get yourself to choke it down. If it's the trouble of actually taking the time to prepare the salad that's holding you back, just buy a ready-made one. Sure, it's more expensive and less healthy, but right now, the point is to make it as easy as possible to keep up the healthy habit.

Only once you've firmly established the habit in its "easy" form, which may take several weeks, should you think about transitioning to a healthier, but more difficult, version of the habit (such as choosing a healthier dressing, in our salad example).

You'll see this theme throughout the book, not just for transitioning to a plant-based diet, and more generally, establishing healthy eating habits, but for starting a fitness program, too.

For now, you can put this knowledge into practice by doing only the amount that's easy for you. This chapter is supposed to be a quick, easy start, and later on I recommend seven different meals to shop for on your next grocery trip. Feel free to work these seven meals into your diet however you like, but err on the side of simple. What I mean is don't say, "I'm changing everything about my diet, today." Instead, gradually incorporate the meals in a way that's exciting and fun, so that your change doesn't feel like a sacrifice.

I recommend working these seven meals into your diet over the course of several weeks. For example, you'll see smoothies recommended as a breakfast option; this doesn't mean you need to (or should) immediately make a smoothie your everyday breakfast. Instead, include it a couple times next week, just enough so that you enjoy it and look forward to next time.

The same goes for the other meals—let's avoid the "cold turkey" approach to getting healthy and going plant-based. I know it works for some people, and if that's absolutely the only way you can get excited about making this change, well, you know yourself better than I do. But if you've never tried to change your habits slowly—an approach that numerous studies about the way the brain works have shown is effective—then you owe it to yourself to at least consider trying this alternative. Although it takes a little longer to build momentum and see results, a slow approach to habit change is the most effective path to real, long-term, automatic change.

With that in mind, let's start!

SIMPLE STEPS FOR ENGINEERING HABITS THAT STICK

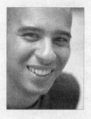

by Leo Babauta
Simplicity blogger, vegan, and author at ZenHabits.net

Trying to stick to a new diet or exercise plan doesn't often work—you can do it for a week or two, but making it last for months or years is nearly impossible unless you focus on changing your habits. The focus for beginners should be on changing habits, not getting quick results.

Unfortunately, most people don't know much about changing habits. This overview is here to make that clearer for you.

Habits are formed when actions are tied to a trigger by consistent repetition so that when the trigger happens, you have an automatic urge to do the action. Some examples:

- When you wake up (trigger), you start the coffee machine (habit).

- When you get to work (trigger), you check your email (habit).

- When you get stressed (trigger), you eat junk food (habit).

Our lives are filled with these trigger-habit combos, often without our being aware of them.

How Did These Habits Form?

They began through consistent repetition over the years. They started with actions performed very consciously at first, before they were a habit, and gradually they became more automatic and less conscious.

If you dislike exercise or are out of shape, then when you exercise, it is painful or unpleasant (negative feedback) and much more comfortable if you don't exercise (positive feedback). If you dislike healthy food, then when you eat healthy food, you think it's boring, bland, or unpleasant (negative feedback), and when you eat unhealthy food, you enjoy yourself more (positive feedback). These feedback loops are what lead to the formation of unhealthy habits. Fortunately, we can reverse the feedback loops by engineering our habit environment:

- **Create positive feedback for the habits you want to form.** Good ways to do this are to start with habits you enjoy and focus on the enjoyment of those habits; create social accountability by telling your friends that you acted on the good habit; and reward yourself.

- **Create negative feedback for not doing the habit.** Social accountability is a good way to do this, too. Tell your friends you're going to act on this new habit for thirty days, and for each day you don't, there will be a negative consequence. For example, you could promise to pay your friend $50 for each day you miss, or, for an even more powerful incentive, donate that money to a charity that you hate.

How to Create a Habit That Lasts in Six Steps

1. Pick only ONE small, positive habit. If your habit is something that can be timed (for example, exercise or meditation), only do it for five or ten minutes at the start. You will expand the time later, but start as small as possible. This is extremely important.

The habit must be performed immediately after a trigger, i.e., something you already do every day. The habit doesn't have to be done at an exact time (seven o'clock in the morning, noon, etc.) but after a specific trigger.

The trigger must be set off every day and exactly once a day. Why every day? If it's not done every day, then you will have a difficult time really forming the habit. Why not more than once a day? We want this to be an easy habit to form—if you have to worry about doing it multiple times a day, the effort it takes to do the habit increases greatly. Let's not start with that barrier.

Also, the habit you choose needs to be specific. It can't be vague. For example, don't say that you want to exercise. Say you want to run for five minutes a day right after you drink coffee in the morning. Don't say you want to drink more water. Say you're going to drink a glass of water when you eat lunch.

If the habit is vague, there's no way to know whether you're doing it. And as such, you'll do it well on some days and not very well on other days.

You should have a measurable change. For example, are you going to do ten push-ups, five minutes of meditation, floss once at night, wake up fifteen minutes earlier, de-clutter ten things from your home a day?

Vague habits fail. Specific ones are likely to succeed.

2. Come up with a plan. Take one week to pick your specific habit (start as small as possible), pick a trigger, plan out how you'll overcome your obstacles, plan who your support network will be, create a log for the habit, pick rewards, and decide what your motivations are. Write down these plans!

3. Do the habit immediately after the trigger for four to six weeks. Build in reminders. Try never to skip doing what you hope to make a habit. The more consistent you are, the stronger the habit will be. What you want to do is create a strong bond between the trigger and the new habit. Each time the trigger happens, you need to perform the new habit. It has to be conscious and deliberate at first, but over time this gets easier, and the new habit becomes almost automatic.

4. Build in positive feedback. Focus on enjoyment, make it a game, create competition, or do it with a partner or group if possible. Here are some good ways to build in positive feedback:

- Enjoy the habit. This is the most effective way. If the habit you want to form is running, do what you can to enjoy the time you spend running—this could mean listening to music, running with a partner, or running on a trail that inspires or relaxes you.

- Announce your success after the habit. After you go for your walk (a new habit), post about it on Facebook, Twitter, or your blog or tell a friend. People congratulate you. You feel great.
- Do something enjoyable immediately after the habit. If you like to check email but want to write for ten minutes a day, check email right after you write for ten minutes (but not before).

5. Report daily to a social group (e.g., blog, Twitter, Facebook, email, or friends at work). Use the group for support when things get difficult. When you feel like not doing the habit, have one or more people you can call on for help. A social group is built-in positive feedback, as well as motivation through accountability. Here are a few notes:

- Find a group you care about. This might be your friends on Facebook or Twitter. It might be your blog readers or members of an online forum. You might have friends, family, or colleagues you can email. Every single time you do the habit, report to the group immediately after. When you're done with your ten-minute run, for example, get into the house, drink a glass of water, and then go to your computer and report it. Or tell your spouse and kids if that's your accountability group.
- If you don't do the habit for some reason, still report it. Commit to reporting either way, no matter what. It will greatly increase your odds of success.

6. Test, adjust, repeat immediately. When you start a habit change, you are testing an approach, and it is very possible it will fail. That's fine. Knowing that your initial approach didn't work is good information, and you should use it to adjust your approach and retry it as soon as possible.

Once you've formed the habit, you are primed for pursuing any future goals. Just remember to start small, increase gradually, and keep it fun.

A Quick-Start Guide to the No Meat Athlete Diet

As I said previously, I want you to start first and start small and only worry about the details once you've started. You only need a few basic pointers at first, and in the next chapter, we'll get on with the nitty-gritty to make sure you're getting all the nourishment you need as a plant-based athlete.

Read this next section and then don't go any further until you've started. Make a few notes, do what it says to choose a few recipes and make a quick list of ingredients, then put the book down, and get yourself to the grocery store.

Healthy Eating Starts with Making Your Own Meals

Perhaps the biggest reason we're so unhealthy these days is because we simply don't cook anymore. We are spending more money than ever on spacious, shiny new kitchens with fancy equipment, but we're not using them—studies show we're eating out for almost half of our meals! And when we do cook, it's rarely any more involved than microwaving a few ingredients or even entire meals that are already prepared (and usually highly processed) for us.

Maybe our lack of cooking is simply the result of our busy, modern lifestyles. Or perhaps it's just a symptom of having so much processed and prepared food available (then again, maybe it's the cause). Either way, we need to get back in the kitchen if we want to get healthy.

The good news is that recipes (and free ones, at that) are everywhere. There are a bunch of plant-based recipes in this book and on my website, www.nomeatathlete.com, to get you started. But they're all over the Web these days, so find a favorite blog from the resources section (page 241), and you'll never again need to stare mindlessly into the fridge wondering what you're going to make tonight.

CHOOSE RECIPES FIRST, THEN GO GROCERY SHOPPING

A lot of people become overwhelmed by the prospect of eating healthier, much less of eliminating meat and other animal products from their diets. It seems like so much work navigating the health food aisle and produce section of the grocery store, spending hours searching for unfamiliar ingredients. And that's before you even think about cooking these strange new foods!

I've got good news: it doesn't have to be nearly this complicated. I've broken down exactly how to get started with a plant-based diet, beginning with seven easy and convenient meals you probably already know how to make. And only *after* you've chosen a few meals and written down the ingredients will you head to the store to shop for exactly what you need (and nothing else).

This approach might sound obvious, but plenty of people do it the other way around—first stocking up on ingredients that seem healthy, then trying to find recipes or come up with meals that match what they have in the fridge. This generally results in a lot of waste and meals that aren't very tasty.

Seven Recipe Staples to Get You Started

You can make almost any recipe healthy simply by starting with mostly unprocessed ingredients. In case you've never done this before and the idea of even choosing recipes (much less changing them) is overwhelming, here's a framework to give your upcoming grocery trip some structure:

1. A smoothie recipe. I recommend working up to starting every day with a smoothie, and a benefit of The Perfect Smoothie Formula (page 106) is that the parts are interchangeable, so you can mix and match ingredients depending on your mood or, more likely, what you've got in the fridge. Start, perhaps, by just swapping out the type of frozen fruit with a different kind than the day before.

2. A salad recipe. Salad is another mini-meal you'll want to have daily. It's pretty easy to throw together a salad without a recipe, but I suspect the reason a lot of people "hate" salads is because they've never made an inspired one. A salad can be so much more than just iceberg lettuce and shredded carrots! Find one that excites you from the salad section (page 98) and put that misconception to bed.

A quick word of warning: be careful with the dressing! Lots of people who eat salads with the best intentions of getting healthy fail to realize that their dressing is so bad it probably turns the whole thing into a net junk food. The good news is that it's simple to make dressing at home, and to make it much healthier than what you can buy in most stores. I'm a big fan of dressing salads with simple lemon juice, extra virgin olive oil, and sea salt.

3. A soup or stew recipe. The great thing about soup is that it's usually easy to make, requiring you to throw some ingredients in a pot to simmer. It's also easy to make a big batch at once, so you can avoid cooking for a day or two if your soup is hearty enough to stand on its own at mealtime. The Hearty Chickpea Pasta Soup (page 98) has become one of my favorites. Pair it, or any other soup or stew you choose, with a hearty roll if you find it doesn't quite fill you up.

4. A veggie burger recipe. Homemade veggie burgers are a thousand times better than frozen store-bought ones. They're also great for freezing so that you'll have something in a pinch when you don't feel like cooking. The Incredible Veggie Burger Formula (page 135) is like the smoothie formula—it provides the skeleton of the recipe and all you've got to do is choose the ingredients you're in the mood for or have on hand.

As for the bun, it's optional. These burgers work on their own, topped with lettuce, salsa, or whatever you like. If you want to have a bun, choose a whole-grain one, or better yet, one made from sprouted grains. And don't forget other options: whole-grain or sprouted-grain pitas are great for Indian or Greek style burgers, and even a large, rolled collard or lettuce leaf can act as a healthy way to hold your burger.

5. A grain, a green, and a bean. This is such a versatile formula for producing a quick, cheap, healthy, and delicious meal. And the best part is that you can cook it in one pot, so clean up is a snap! Make it from a recipe like the Hawaiian Beans and Rice (page 134) first and then experiment with others on your own. How about some adzuki beans, quinoa, bok choy, and Perfect Peanut Sauce (page 147)? Kidney beans, collard greens, and millet (with hot sauce!)? The possibilities are endless and so very simple.

6. Burrito and taco recipes. I've included these because I know they're a favorite of the college or twenty-something chef for their simplicity and deliciousness. But I like them because they're a great vehicle for raw vegetables—you can cook the main filling, but then top it with fresh tomatoes, jalapenos, lettuce, cilantro, lime juice, avocado, and anything else you like.

Mexican Green Chile Beans and Rice (page 132) is a delicious recipe to start with as the base for your tacos or burritos. Pile them with fresh tomatoes, avocado, salsa, and lime juice and serve in soft corn tortillas for some authenticity—or, if you want bonus points, wrap your burritos in large collard or kale leaves.

7. A pasta dish. You'll start to notice something after you've planned and cooked a few plant-based meals from this book or elsewhere: almost every meal is a one-dish wonder. Rather than having a main dish and two or three sides, like a traditional (well, Western) meal, you'll very often eat just one dish that takes up the entire plate or bowl.

I have a theory about why this is. In a traditional American diet, the food in the center of the plate is meat—a source of protein, perhaps with some fat. The side dishes, often a starch and a vegetable, are your carbohydrates. With plant-based food though, there aren't as many options for efficient sources of protein: although you can get plenty of "the big P" from beans, veggies, nuts, and grains, these foods generally pack more than just protein (often complex carbohydrates and healthy, monounsaturated fats). If you were to add carbohydrate-rich side dishes to an already carbo-rich main dish, the meal would become unbalanced. And so we incorporate everything into one delicious dish, attempting to achieve a balanced mix of protein, fat, and carbohydrates.

And here's where pasta shines, if you choose your noodles well and don't overdo it on the portion size. It's a one-dish meal that fits right into a plant-based diet, without seeming overly foreign to long-time omnivores. I'm a big fan of using quinoa pasta to increase the nutrition a little bit, but if you want to save money (or just keep it as "normal" as possible while you're transitioning to this diet), choose a whole-wheat or multigrain blend.

A Healthy Eater's Guide to the Grocery Store

The recipe staples I've listed are based on whole, fresh ingredients, so you probably won't need to do much substituting if you're using the recipes in this book to make them. But I hope you'll choose some other recipes as well, and in some cases, you will need to change out ingredients for healthier alternatives. Here are some basics to keep in mind when you go shopping for food.

Fresh Produce: One Aisle of the Store, More than Half of Your Groceries

You know you're doing well if you spend about two-thirds to three-quarters of your shopping time and money in the fresh produce section. You can't go wrong here, as long as most of what you're getting isn't in packages.

Should you go organic? If you've got the budget for it, sure, but you can stretch your dollar by getting organic varieties of only the "dirty dozen," the foods listed each year by the Environmental Working Group (www.ewg.org/foodnews) as the most pesticide-laden conventionally farmed foods.

As for your choice of leafy greens, generally the darker varieties pack the greatest nutritional punch. Although I think the currently fashionable slamming of iceberg lettuce is a little unfair, it's good to mix it up with some darker, more vitamin-rich leafy greens like arugula, spinach, kale, collards, or even simply romaine.

In the fruit section, grab a mix of fruits that you'll enjoy snacking on or even eating after a meal for dessert.

When you can, buy produce that's local. (A farmers market is a better bet for this than the store.) This way you'll be less likely to get mass-produced, pale, vitamin- and nutrient-devoid stand-ins for the real thing. Fruits and vegetables lose a lot of their nutritional goodness within a few days of being picked, so the closer to the source and the less time your food spends in the back of a truck, the better.

THE (UNINTENTIONAL) VEGAN MARATHONER

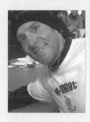

By Tom Giammalvo

I used to watch lots of TV, play video games into the wee hours of the morning, smoke, work nights, and not care about what I ate. I changed by taking small steps. I am now a marathoner, trail runner, cyclist, triathlete, active member of National Ski Patrol, active member of the Greater New Bedford (Massachusetts) Track Club, and most importantly, a no-meat athlete!

My journey began in 2010 when, ready for a change from a mostly-sedentary life filled with cigarettes and energy drinks, I completed the P90x program, a ninety-day home exercise and nutrition program by Beach Body. I completed my first 5K run in 2010, in 28:39.

Influenced by my godchildren, I decided to quit smoking and opt for a healthier lifestyle. There is a book called the *Accidental Vegan*, and I feel I could label myself as such. I never intended to go vegan, but as my running improved, I looked for a greater edge, and healthy eating was working. I gradually transitioned to a vegan diet, first cutting out red meat, then chicken, then fish, and finally dairy products.

I found as I turned to a vegan lifestyle, my recovery after runs improved, and I needed fewer Ace wraps following hard workouts. I trained from November through March and crossed the finish line of the New Bedford Half Marathon in 1:45:45 as a no-meat athlete. I wanted more, and in October 2011, I finished the Cape Cod Marathon with a time of 3:48:10.

My journey had just begun, and in the next two years, I ran another half marathon, another marathon, and even my first ultramarathon!

Through my first months of transformation, I noticed an improved sense of overall well-being and didn't experience the tired feeling you normally get after eating a typical meal on the standard Western diet. I haven't been sick since going vegan. The environmental benefits and benefits to animals are, for me, just icing on the cake!

In the last two years I've become stronger, influenced others, met some amazing plant-based eaters along the way, and lived a rewarding no-meat athlete lifestyle. I encourage anyone to give it a try.

IF YOU CAN'T GET IT FRESH, GO FOR FROZEN

If fresh, local produce isn't an option, isn't convenient, or just isn't in your budget (I hear you!), don't hesitate to buy and use frozen fruits and vegetables. They're picked and frozen when perfectly ripe, so they are very high in nutrients, even after being frozen and thawed. Even better, they're low-cost, easy to store and use, and perfect for days when you're extra busy and haven't had a chance to pick up fresh produce.

Grains: They're Nothing to Fear, but Don't Go Overboard

Recently there's been a strong low-carb, anti-grain (and especially anti-wheat) vibe in the health community, in part because of the popularity of the Paleo diet. I'm still on board the grain train, but I agree with my friend and coauthor, Matthew Ruscigno, that although we don't need to banish grains from our pantries, most people eat too much of them, especially wheat, which is so common in even health-conscious eaters' diets.

If you're not careful, it's easy to eat some form of wheat in every single one of your meals—in the form of bagels, cereal, pasta, bread, snacks, and desserts. Don't do that. Remember, variety in diet is one of the keys to ensuring we don't become deficient in any one nutrient, vitamin, or mineral, so to eat any single food so often (when there are hundreds at our disposal) simply doesn't make sense.

Variety in diet is one of the keys to ensuring we don't become deficient in any one nutrient, vitamin, or mineral.

As long as you don't have a wheat allergy or Celiac disease, it's fine to eat wheat now and then—just not with every meal. Instead, round out your dishes with grains other than wheat or with healthier pseudograins like quinoa, which is technically a seed. When you do buy grains, get whole-grain, brown, or sprouted-grain versions, rather than refined whites, which have been stripped of many nutrients and the fiber that serves to tell you that you're full.

And know that most any grain or pseudograin can stand in for any other in a basic recipe. Don't be afraid to mix things up with alternatives like quinoa, amaranth, buckwheat, millet (all pseudograins), barley, or even spelt and bulgur, which are ancient forms of wheat with different nutrient profiles from the modern version. The same goes for flours made from any of these.

Oils: When It Comes to Controversy, Go for Compromise

There's a lot of argument over the best oil to use in your cooking. In fact, many respected health professionals, such as physician and nutrition expert John McDougall, M.D., advocate consuming no oil, because, after all, it's not a whole food.

I take a slightly less extreme approach and believe that when chosen carefully and used sparingly, oils can help plant-based athletes increase their caloric intake and improve performance. Brendan Brazier and Scott Jurek, two of the best-known and most accomplished of such athletes, both advocate certain oils for their performance and health benefits, as does Walter Willett, M.D., chairman of the department of nutrition at the Harvard School of Public Health and author of several books on nutrition.

WHEN OIL CAN'T STAND THE HEAT

The primary benefits of most plant-based oils are their fat profiles. With a few exceptions, these oils are high in healthy, monounsaturated fats that are not greatly altered by heat so long as they're not heated above their smoke points—the temperature at which a given oil begins to break down, its flavor and nutritional benefits degrade, and it begins to smoke.

Though technically some vitamins and minerals are lost at even low cooking temperatures, oil contains few of these to begin with, so it's no great loss to heat them below their smoke points, at which their healthy fats remain intact.

Personally, I use olive oil for salads and some low-temperature cooking, coconut oil for other low-temperature cooking and in smoothies or as a butter substitute on toast or popcorn, and grapeseed oil for cooking at higher temperatures. Watch out for highly processed and heated oils, such as the most nondescript of all, vegetable oil.

Whichever oil you choose, go easy on it: don't use a tablespoon when a teaspoon will do. It's not a whole food, it packs a lot of calories into a very small space, and it loses a lot of its nutritional value when heated.

Condiments and Processed Snacks: Check Ingredients and Consume in Moderation

As long as you're consuming condiments in relatively small quantities, I see no problem with continuing to eat most of the ones you enjoy.

The big rule here is to check out the ingredients list and make sure you recognize them all and that as many as possible are whole foods. Look out for high-fructose corn syrup, which is anything but whole, and appears in countless condiments. And look out for oils here—many condiments use low-quality oils that you'll want to avoid. Check the sodium content, too, because prepared foods can be the source of a huge amount of salt. Preparing condiments yourself will help tremendously, so find recipes for salsa, hummus, baba ganoush, barbecue sauce, and others.

While we're on the topic of salt, don't go crazy with it. According to Joel Fuhrman, M.D., for millions of years humans did not add any salt to their food. The sodium naturally present in foods amounts to only 600–800 mg per day, while even a half teaspoon of salt packs close to 1,000 mg of sodium. Keep in mind, however, that iodized table salt is a major source of iodine for many Americans, so if you're going to limit salt or use non-iodized sea salt, consider supplementing as very few foods contain iodine naturally.

For snacks, the same principles apply: look at the ingredients and make sure they're whole foods and watch out for salt and processed oils. Raw or roasted nuts are the best thing you'll find in the snack aisle.

Drinks: One Aisle to Skip, with a Few Exceptions

There's almost nothing worth buying in the beverage aisle of the grocery store. Mostly what you'll find there is no more than sweetened, colored, and carbonated water. (Coconut water and some natural sports drinks are useful for replenishing glycogen stores during long workouts and races, which we'll talk about later, but not as an everyday calorie source.)

Drink water. If that's boring, add some lemon or lime juice. You'll eventually get used to it. Tea is good, too, and if you're going to drink caffeine, it's far gentler on your body than coffee. Green tea is a favorite of mine. But there are also a huge variety of herbal teas that are naturally caffeine-free, and they're delicious and packed full of antioxidants. If you're new to tea, I recommend lightly sweetening it at first with a few drops of agave nectar and gradually reducing the amount of agave you use until you enjoy the taste of tea by itself.

Ten Simple Food Rules of the No Meat Athlete Diet

The more I learn about habits, the more I believe that simplicity is the best policy—especially when it comes to food.

I'm not a fan of restrictions or numbers when it's time to eat. Food, and the time we spend eating it, should be enjoyed—it's one of the great pleasures of life, and to constrain it with complicated rules and numbers is completely unnatural.

Simplicity is the reason author Michael Pollan's three-sentence manifesto from *In Defense of Food* has resonated so well. ("Eat food. Mostly plants. Not too much.") And the stickiness of that phrase is probably what led Pollan to write *Food Rules*, another goodie full of short, memorable rules of thumb like, "Eat only what your great-grandmother would recognize as food."

Here, I list the simple food rules I live by. They're not meant to be as catchy or easy to remember as Pollan's, but they're an honest distillation of what I believe is the healthiest way to eat. Not just this month or until you lose those last fifteen pounds, but for life.

1. Avoid processed foods and choose whole, unrefined foods instead.

This one should come as no surprise. It's listed first because if you were to throw out every other message you've heard about healthy food and retain only the three words "eat whole foods," you would dramatically improve the way you eat if you're currently doing something different.

But this single guideline flies in the face of the way people eat in the Western world today, so you'll have to reject the shiny pseudo-food that food manufacturers want you to buy. Some specific examples of what you're looking for:

- ▸ Brown rice instead of white
- ▸ Fruits instead of fruit juice
- ▸ Whole-fruit smoothies instead of juice that's been separated from the fiber
- ▸ Whole-wheat flour instead of white (more on wheat in a bit)

2. Get most of your food from plants.

Unlike many other vegetarians and vegans, I tend not to believe that meat and eggs are inherently bad for you (dairy products are a different story—to me, drinking milk from another species and beyond infancy doesn't make any sense). We've seen that people can thrive on a variety of omnivorous and plant-based diets, and I think we're built to handle either one pretty well.

The problem with meat, as far as health goes, is the sheer amount most people consume. Although our ancestors might have gone several days between successful hunts and the meat that resulted, modern people treat every meal like a post-hunt feast. The caloric density of that much meat leaves little room for other foods and puts a digestive load on our bodies that leaves us feeling sluggish and full for hours after big meals.

People in many countries other than the United States use meat as a flavoring agent or as a side dish, perhaps, but rarely as the focus of the meal. I believe that if the ethical implications don't bother you and you're going to continue to eat meat, this is the only healthy way to do it.

3. Cook your own food.

To follow the first guideline of eating whole foods nearly dictates that you prepare your own food. Nonetheless, I've included it as its own rule because it runs counter to the way so many people now obtain their meals.

Much of Section I of this book is dedicated to helping you make your way into the kitchen and start cooking. But it doesn't stop with preparing meals: just about any food worth eating can be prepared at home, bringing you one step closer to the source of the food you eat and giving you complete knowledge of every single ingredient that goes into it.

Here are a few foods you might be tempted to buy that you can make at home with equipment no more sophisticated than a food processor or high-speed blender.

- ▶ Hummus
- ▶ Baba ganoush
- ▶ Pesto
- ▶ Sauces: tomato, barbecue, and ketchup
- ▶ Nut butters
- ▶ Flour from grains or beans
- ▶ Sprouts
- ▶ Smoothies
- ▶ Sports drinks

4. Make raw fruits and vegetables a big part of your diet.

There's a lot of debate over the virtues of raw versus cooked food. On one hand, some say that raw food is more easily digested because digestive enzymes that exist in the raw state are denatured by excessive heat. On the other hand, many foods are inedible unless they are cooked, and cooking is a practice that has gone on for much of our existence (long enough to have influenced our evolution).

I take the middle ground on this one, choosing to eat foods in both states. But because we're so used to eating cooked foods, it's only raw foods that we need to make a conscious effort to make sure we eat each day.

RAW VEGGIES ARE GREAT, BUT SOMETIMES IT PAYS TO COOK THEM

Cooking can improve the nutritional profile of some vegetables. For example, cooking carrots actually increases the amount of beta-carotene that our bodies can absorb. The same is true for tomatoes—cooking breaks down the fibrous walls and increases the availability of the phytochemical lycopene. Early studies show that lycopene may be involved in the prevention of cancer. There's still a lot to learn, but the research is promising.

One of the best habits you can develop is having a mostly-raw smoothie each morning and a big salad each afternoon. Combine this with a few pieces of fresh fruit for snacks throughout the day, and you're getting a significant amount of wholesome, raw food without even thinking about it. Which brings me to the next guideline.

5. Drink a smoothie and eat a salad every single day.

Even if you ate whatever you wanted the rest of the day, I'd be willing to bet you wouldn't get fat as long as you made sure to drink a smoothie and eat a big salad every single day.

Sure, if you were to eat at McDonald's for lunch and Outback Steakhouse for dinner the rest of the time, you could probably succeed at packing on a few pounds. But here's the thing: The smoothie and salad act as anchors that keep you on track, to remind you just how great it feels to put real, fresh fruits and vegetables in your body. After you start the day with a smoothie, McDonald's for lunch doesn't seem so good anymore. And when it's time to start thinking about dinner, the salad is there to help you make a good choice.

In this way, those two healthy meals turn into three or four—which doesn't leave much room for junk.

6. Don't eat too much wheat (or any one food, really!).

I realize that you might have no desire to stop eating bread and wheat pasta. And that's fine. I don't either.

But so many food products in our culture are now based on wheat that it's very easy for it to show up in *every single meal* you eat if you don't pay attention! Relying so heavily on a single food just doesn't make much sense, even before you consider the reasons many top athletes now avoid wheat.

People have varying levels of sensitivity to wheat. For some people, gluten is tremendously difficult to digest. For others, the sensitivity isn't so severe that it's recognized as a problem, but wheat nevertheless may adversely affect their energy levels. Health problems associated with gluten occur even with 100 percent whole wheat products, not just refined wheat flour (which most athletes avoid anyway, except perhaps at certain key times around workouts).

The good news is that there are now plenty of good alternatives to wheat products, especially when it comes to pasta, the runners' staple. Among the many varieties are those made from rice, quinoa, and even chickpea flour.

My suggestion: Don't cut out wheat completely if you don't have a gluten sensitivity, but limit it to one meal a day instead of three or four, or ideally to just a few meals a week, like any other food.

7. Eat a wide variety of foods.

If the idea of eating a mostly vegetarian diet doesn't appeal to you, it's likely that you view it as a "taking away" process. Maybe your meals are centered around meat, and without it, the plate would seem pretty empty.

But the reality is quite different than that. If you're mindful of what you eat and don't simply rely on vegetarian junk food, you'll actually end up *adding* many foods to your diet as you're forced to go outside of your normal routine and explore new options at home and in restaurants.

This is a great thing for your health. It means you'll get a broad mix of vitamins and minerals, rather than potentially getting way more than you need of certain ones and none of many others, as you might if you were to eat the same few foods over and over.

8. With the exception of a daily smoothie, don't drink your calories.

If you've paid any attention to healthy eating over the past few years, this guideline probably isn't new to you. It's essentially a restatement of the "eat whole foods" guideline because most drinks with substantial amounts of calories are processed.

Because drinks, even fruit juices, take up relatively little room in your stomach, it's very easy to take in way too many calories before you feel full.

This reasoning applies to smoothies as well because you can drink much more fruit when it's blended into a smoothie than you could eat whole. But as long as they're made with whole ingredients, I give them a pass because they're such a great way to start the day with a bunch of fresh fruits and vegetables.

But please, do whatever it takes to stop drinking soda, even diet soda. It's caffeinated sugar water—or fake-sugar water, perhaps worse—and it has no place in a healthy diet. The same goes for most commercial energy drinks and sports drinks. Although sugary sports drinks have a place in an athlete's diet—during long workouts, when you need to replenish carbohydrate reserves in your blood—there's simply no reason to take in that much sugar at other times.

> *Do whatever it takes to stop drinking soda, even diet soda. It has no place in a healthy diet.*

9. Eat when you're hungry, but make sure you really are hungry.

Eating is one of the true joys in our lives, and to me, imposing a limit on our intake significantly takes away from that. Fortunately, if you're eating the right foods, limiting your intake is unnecessary unless you've got a serious weight problem. As we've mentioned several times now, when you eat foods that contain all of their original nutrients and are in a form close to their natural one, your body will naturally feel full at the right time. The stretch and density receptors in your stomach tell your brain that you've had enough for now and additional intake will become uncomfortable.

That is, if you give your body a chance to realize you're full. Rushing through your meals sidesteps the system, allowing you to take in excess food before your stomach has had a chance to sense fullness. Take your time, chew your food, and pay attention to how you feel.

The Japanese have a phrase *hara hachi bu*, which refers to the practice of eating only until you are 80 percent full. It works well because there's a lag time between when you eat a food and when you feel its volume in your stomach. Start paying attention to how full you feel, and use that as an indicator of when you should stop eating instead of waiting until your plate is clean or the sitcom is over.

10. Break some of these rules from time to time.

To me, this guideline is crucial. Especially if you're new to eating healthfully, the idea of "I can never eat [blank] again" is poison to your long-term goals.

I'm not saying you should break all of them. Some, such as eating only plant foods, may carry with them an ethical obligation for you, in which case you probably won't wish to break them ever.

But other than that, I think being flexible in your approach to food is healthier and better for your entire being than forcing yourself to be overly restrictive at every meal. Break a few of these rules when the time is right. For some people, like *The 4-Hour Body* author Tim Ferriss, that means having a "cheat day" once a week where you can eat literally any food you want and being uber-strict the rest of the time. If such extremes don't work for you, find an alternative plan for allowing yourself to occasionally zig instead of zag.

Best of all, strive to reach the point where you don't need a plan—indulge when the rare situation arises, knowing that your healthy way of eating is so ingrained that you're not at risk for "falling off the wagon" because of a single transgression.

> *If you're new to eating healthfully, the idea of "I can never eat [blank] again" is poison to your long-term goals.*

TAKING YOUR (PLANT-BASED) SHOW ON THE ROAD

Of all the inconveniences of being vegan in a non-vegan world, travel just might be the toughest to deal with.

Sure, you could grab a burger on the go. People with otherwise healthy diets do it all the time, maybe a couple times a month or more. And if you don't have an ethical connection to your plant-based diet, there's no reason you couldn't, too. The funny thing is, though, I bet that won't happen.

"Plant-based" is a label people take seriously, much more so than "healthy." It feels wrong to tell people you're a vegan when just three days ago you knocked back a burger and a milkshake because there weren't any other options. Maybe on another healthy diet, but not a vegan one.

And that's the thing. Others make exceptions. You prepare.

What can you bring along to fill you up? Depending on the circumstances of your travel (Is it by car or plane? Is there a kitchen in your hotel? Is there a health-food store nearby, or are you in the middle of nowhere?), I recommend the following:

- A bag of nuts or trail mix
- A few pieces of fruit, or even a full bunch of bananas if that's all you can find
- Dried fruit—buy it or get a dehydrator and make it yourself
- Hummus (perhaps homemade) in a pita
- A bagel or pita with nut butter (again, homemade is a possibility)
- Carrots, celery, broccoli, or any other chopped vegetable and something like hummus to dip it in
- A meal replacement powder, like Vega One, mixed in a shaker cup with water, almond milk, or another drink you've got on hand

What about Eating Out?

I asked several pro athletes, cookbook authors, and vegan bloggers how they survive when they're on the road, and the most common answer they came up with was *Happy Cow*. That's www.happycow.net, a website that happens to be the best resource, bar none, for finding vegetarian- and vegan-friendly restaurants while you're on the road.

How to Get from Here to Plant-Based

As you can probably guess by now, my suggestion for transitioning to a plant-based diet is to do it gradually. Again, there are people for whom the all-or-nothing approach works. And I get it—it's exciting and motivating to think that from this day forward, things are going to be different. But think for a minute about other times you've attempted to change that way, whether it was a diet or a New Year's resolution or something else. If you can think of more than a few times when that approach has failed to create lasting change, I'm asking you to try going about it differently.

I made two attempts to go vegetarian. The first failed miserably after a week; the second has lasted four and a half years, has increased in intensity (I became vegan after two years), and I have no plans to go back.

From those two experiences, and from what I've seen others experience, here's what I think are the most important keys to making the change last.

1. At first, don't try to "never eat meat again."

I have nothing but admiration for those who can give up meat, once and for all, right off the bat. They decide, right away, that they're going vegetarian or even vegan, and they never go back.

I wish I could say it worked like that for me. Instead, for that entire first week of my failed attempt, I just kept thinking about how hard it was, that there was no way I could actually make my vegetarian foray last.

What was different about the second time, when the change lasted? A lot of factors, a big one being that I set end-dates. At first, I said I'd eat vegetarian and fish for ten days. After that, I could go back if I wanted. But I liked how I felt, so the next time, I set the mark at thirty days and started cutting out the fish, too. Again, if I got to the end and decided to quit, it was cool. In this way, by the time I started thinking, "I'll never eat meat again," I didn't really like eating meat anymore. Or at least I was accustomed to not eating it. And so it never felt like much of a sacrifice.

2. Transition smoothly, from four legs to two legs to no legs.

Making drastic changes is fun, exciting, and sometimes effective. For me, it wasn't. That first time, I just stopped eating all meat. It didn't last.

The second time, I stopped eating four-legged animals (red meat and pork) first *for an entire year.* It wasn't part of a plan to go vegetarian; I just felt at the time that because eating vegetarian was too hard for me, this was the next best thing.

It was easy to get by on turkey burgers, seafood, and lots of chicken. And all the Italian recipes I loved to cook worked just fine when I replaced the ground lamb, pork, or beef with birds, so it was pretty easy.

START WHERE YOU ARE

Another trick for gradually transitioning is to "start where you are," which means eat more of the plant-based meals you like and make slight changes to your meals with meat to slowly phase it out. For example, if you like cooking beef and broccoli, you can use a higher proportion of broccoli each time until the meal is mostly broccoli and almost no beef.

Then, when I decided I wanted to go further, I cut out our two-legged flying feathered friends. I still ate fish for a few weeks, unsure whether I wanted to go all the way. Then one day, I realized that I didn't really like eating fish anymore. By that time, I ate so little of it that I don't even remember when I "officially" stopped. And it wasn't until two years later, after gradually phasing out dairy, that I decided to become vegan.

It was all so easy. I've since learned that making tiny changes, stacked on top of each other, is the most effective way to make big changes. That's how I recommend you do it.

3. Plan for each new phase.

If you decide on the spur of the moment to change, you'll likely fail like I did the first time. So how exactly does one plan to give up chicken, for example? First, you make sure you don't have chicken in your house. Finish it up or give it away. Then do a little research. Because you'll be cutting out a protein source, make sure you don't just replace it with carbohydrates. Pick out a few hearty, healthy vegetarian meals you can try, like the ones in this book.

Next, you plan an entire week's worth of meals that don't include chicken. Pick a few vegetarian recipes (the ones suggested earlier in this chapter are a great place to start), perhaps even a few with "meatless" chicken (made from soy or other vegetarian protein substitutes) while you adjust. Then go to the grocery store to get what you need for the week and enjoy the progress you're making and the way you feel as your diet changes.

And don't forget: if you're going on a car trip, or maybe to a party where they won't have anything you eat, be prepared. Get some snacks or even eat a small meal beforehand so that you won't have to rely on willpower to get you through it.

4. Give yourself a break!

I don't mean a break from vegetarianism, I mean let yourself eat some less-than-ideal foods to make the changes easier.

When you first cut out meat, let yourself eat some extra pasta, fake meats, or even cheese. Sure, none of these are great for you, but the point is to ease the shock and make the transition more pleasant so that you aren't tempted to quit.

I still eat vegan sausage from time to time when I'm really craving it. It's made from wheat gluten, and I don't pretend that it's a whole food or really great for me. But if it takes an occasional splurge to eat a diet that, the other 95 percent of the time, compels me to make better choices, then to me, that's worth it.

5. Try new foods.

The most exciting part of a plant-based diet is all the new foods there are to experience. Sure, you could have tried them all along, but for some reason you didn't when it was easy to fill the plate with meat, potatoes, and when you were feeling really saucy, a vegetable.

Take advantage of a new reason to expand your horizons. Make some Indian food, go to a Thai restaurant, or eat Ethiopian food with your hands. Find a weird-looking, brown, hairy root in the produce section of the grocery store and search for "recipes based on weird-looking, brown, hairy roots" on the Internet and make one of them. (Make sure you catch the name of said root because I promise the cashier will not know it.)

Allowing yourself to experience all these new flavors and textures will take your attention off of what's missing from your plate and shift it to what's new and interesting. In short: relax your expectations and make it easy on yourself.

Trust me, I know how hard it is when you're all pumped up to make a big change to understand that your willpower and enthusiasm will, at some point, wane. Rather than crashing at that point and feeling like you failed, I've learned that you're so much more likely to succeed if you don't expect too much of yourself.

Go slowly, go smoothly, and don't beat yourself up over mistakes. And when you've got questions or concerns, reach out. It's not hard to find someone who wants you to be vegetarian and would be happy to help.

"This All Sounds Good, but I Need Specifics."

What I've outlined in this chapter represents 80 percent of the story of what a plant-based diet for athletes looks like: simple, easy-to-follow guidelines and a relatively laid-back, natural approach to eating. But it's not quite the entire picture.

I'd be lying if I said there wasn't a little more than this. The first thing most people ask when I tell them I'm an ultramarathoner and a vegan is, you guessed it, "Where do you get your protein?" Although it's not the big deal most people make it out to be, protein is something to consider, so we'll get into how much protein (and other nutrients) you need and some easy ways to make sure your diet is balanced. We also haven't yet touched on iron or B_{12}, two other deficiencies in some people's plant-based diets that we'll need to make sure aren't an issue for you.

In the next chapter, we'll get into all of this. But for now, the important thing is to start.

CHAPTER 3

PLANT-BASED NUTRITION FOR SPORTS: AN IN-DEPTH GUIDE

To put plant-based nutrition for athletes on a more solid foundation than I ever could, I asked Matthew Ruscigno, M.P.H., R.D., who is vegan and has served as chairman of the Vegetarian Nutrition Practice Group of the Academy of Nutrition and Dietetics, to write this chapter, the most in-depth section about nutrition in the book. But don't think that Matt's just a dietitian who doesn't know about what it's like to be an athlete; among other endeavors, he's an ultra-distance cyclist who has placed tenth in the Furnace Creek 508, a 508-mile solo bike race through Death Valley. You're in good hands.

—Matt Frazier

These days, there is so much nutrition information available, it isn't easy to discern what's best for you. And the stakes are high! Diet plays a key role in how we feel and perform, as well as in long-term disease prevention.

The main theme of this chapter is that plant-based nutrition doesn't rely only on specific foods for specific nutrients, contrary to what we've been taught and to conventional wisdom. You probably grew up learning that milk is the best source for calcium and that meat is the best source of protein because of very successful advertising campaigns associated with these foods. These campaigns were so effective that people now confuse food with nutrients. It's such a pervasive idea that even proponents of plant-based diets sometimes fall into this trap and compare soymilk directly to dairy milk, or beans directly to meat, to prove their nutritional value.

But there's no need to make these comparisons. Why? Because in plant-based nutrition, the focus is on eating a variety of whole foods that contain many nutrients in varying amounts. We don't need to get 30 percent of our calcium from any single source because we can get calcium from half a dozen different sources.

This chapter covers the basics of plant-based nutrition to give you the confidence to prepare and eat vegan and vegetarian meals. Chapters 8 and 9 have additional information on training techniques and how to eat around your workouts.

The Benefits of Getting Nutrients from a Variety of Sources

Plant-based whole foods are incredibly rich sources of the vitamins and minerals we need. Traditional nutrition information assumes that people eat only small amounts of fresh fruits, vegetables, or whole grains. In plant-based nutrition, the emphasis is on variety and significant amounts of these nutrient-dense foods. This variety is beneficial for our taste buds and is the basis of a solid nutrition plan that will meet your needs. As you learn more about plant-based nutrition, consider the following key points:

1. You absorb more nutrients when you consume them in smaller amounts. Your body is not an empty bucket that collects extra nutrients. It only absorbs and uses the nutrients it needs at the time; if you eat more than needed, your body discards them. For example, if you take an 18 mg iron supplement all at once, it will be poorly absorbed. Iron absorption is highest when only small amounts are consumed at one time. This is true for most nutrients.

2. When you have variety in your diet, you have more opportunities to get the nutrients you need. The average person's diet has very little variety. When you eat only a few types of foods, you have fewer opportunities to get the nutrients you need. In plant-based nutrition, the emphasis is on variety because there are so many nutrient-dense plant foods.

In plant-based nutrition, the emphasis is on variety because there are so many nutrient-dense plant foods.

For example, what if you don't want to consume dairy products? Does that mean you'll be lacking in calcium? Of course not. You can get calcium from kale, broccoli, collard greens, and tofu, among other foods. Don't like leafy greens? Then there's soymilk. Don't like soymilk? Try almond milk. Once you open the door to variety, your opportunities to get the nutrients you need are near limitless.

3. A varied diet acts as insurance against nutritional deficiency. On one hand, if you eat the same ten foods day after day, week after week, there's a chance you'll eventually become deficient in a certain amino acid, vitamin, or nutrient that happens to be lacking from that small selection of foods. On the other hand, if you eat a huge variety of whole foods each week, it's far less likely that you'll be missing any specific nutrient for long.

DON'T BE MISLED BY SMALL SERVING SIZES

If you look at the nutrition facts for fruits and vegetables, you may be surprised to see very low numbers. Why? Because the serving sizes of these foods are small compared to what plant-based athletes eat.

The serving size for cooked broccoli is only half of a cup (36 g). That's only a few florets! When broccoli becomes the focus of your dinner, it's easy and reasonable to eat three cups (213 g), especially if you're adding it to a stir-fry, where vegetables cook down when heated thoroughly. In those three cups (213 g) of broccoli, you get six servings and six times the nutrients you would if you were to eat only one serving. This adds up to 10 percent of the daily requirement for calcium and iron in only sixty calories.

The same is true with fruit. My favorite breakfast is mashed up bananas with almond butter and diced apples. I use four ripe bananas or even more when I have a hard training day ahead. Bananas are mostly carbohydrate, but in four servings, you get five grams of protein. Not enough to recommend bananas as a source of protein, but it is slightly more than the amount of protein in one small egg!

Macronutrients: Getting the Calories You Need from Carbohydrate, Protein, and Fat

There's a scene in the terrific documentary *Super Size Me* in which people on the street are asked what they think a calorie is. The responses are mostly about how they are bad for you or that they should be avoided. This scene demonstrates just how confused most people are when it comes to nutrition.

Calories are nothing more than units of measure for energy—they're neither good nor bad until we view them in a particular context. Calories are found in all foods in the form of carbohydrate, protein, or fat. Collectively, these sources of calories are called macronutrients; they always have calories and are the *only* sources of calories.

Below, I've outlined how carbohydrates are the absolute best source of fuel for your workouts, how plant protein is more than adequate, and how fat in a plant-based diet is both essential and beneficial. I want you to understand this information well to be the best athlete possible and a smart advocate for vegetarian or vegan eating.

CALCULATING YOUR DAILY CALORIES

Although it's not absolutely necessary to figure out your ideal daily intake of total calories or how this number breaks down into carbohydrate, protein, and fat components, it is worthwhile for serious athletes (and control freaks and nerds, like us).

Use the method below to determine your daily caloric needs with the caveat that it's only an estimate because of variables, including lean body mass, fitness level, and metabolism rate. For a more accurate assessment, your caloric needs can be measured through direct or indirect calorimetry in a laboratory.

Step 1: First, we need to calculate your Basal Metabolic Rate (BMR) using your weight, height, and age. BMR calculates the number of daily calories you would need to sustain life if you were totally immobile; i.e., it's the energy required just to stay alive!

Women: BMR = 655 + (4.35 x weight in pounds) + (4.7 x height in inches) - (4.7 x age in years)

Men: BMR = 66 + (6.23 x weight in pounds) + (12.7 x height in inches) - (6.8 x age in years)

Step 2: Next we use the Harris-Benedict Formula to multiply your BMR by the appropriate physical activity factor. If you are:

- **Sedentary** (little or no exercise): BMR x 1.2 = total calories needed per day
- **Lightly active** (light exercise/sports 1 to 3 days/week): BMR x 1.375 = total calories needed per day
- **Moderately active** (moderate exercise/sports 3 to 5 days/week): BMR x 1.55 = total calories needed per day
- **Very active** (hard exercise/sports 6 to 7 days a week): BMR x 1.725 = total calories needed per day
- **Extremely active** (very hard exercise/sports and physical job or training twice a day): BMR x 1.9 = total calories needed per day

The question is can you get all of the calories you need from plants? Be assured that you can, easily. For example, Chris Carmichael, the famous

(continued)

cycling coach, recommends in his book *Food For Fitness* that athletes get roughly 65 percent of their caloric intake from carbohydrate, 13 percent from protein, and 22 percent from fat. His numbers are not unique and can be easily met with a plant-based diet. Visit www.nomeatathlete.com/calculations for precise instructions on how to calculate these percentages in terms of grams of each macronutrient.

Carmichael's guidelines vary based on specific training, as do mine, but not by much. One of the most common mistakes I find when consulting with plant-based athletes is they are not consuming enough calories to fuel their workouts. To build muscle, reduce fatigue, and get the most out of your workouts, you have to take in enough energy through the food you eat.

Carbohydrate: Make It Your Fuel of Choice

Carbohydrate is the calorie that's most readily turned to energy to fuel our activities. Research shows that carbohydrate, which closely resembles the glucose and glycogen our cells use for energy, helps athletes perform their best and should be the base of a healthy diet for active people.

Carbohydrates break down into two groups: complex and simple. Complex carbohydrates are long chains of glucose found in the starch and cellulose of plants. In addition to being a preferred fuel source, complex carbohydrates are a rich source of fiber. Complex carbohydrates are the fuel of choice for athletes, and plant foods like whole grains, starchy vegetables, and legumes are high in complex carbohydrates.

Simple carbohydrates are those found in fruits and refined wheat and sugar products. They are short-chain molecules and are very rapidly digested and turned to energy.

Between 50 and 70 percent of your calories should be from carbohydrates. Starchy vegetables and whole grains are the most nutritional sources of complex carbohydrates. Legumes also contain significant amounts of carbohydrate, which should be taken into consideration when building meals.

Choose the Right Carbs for Energy

From the Atkins to the Paleo diet, it seems like many people are avoiding carbs these days. And the most confusing part is that people who actively reduce their carbohydrate intake appear to lose weight, get strong, and feel healthier. Why is that?

A common thread among low-carb diet plans is that they considerably reduce or eliminate refined carbohydrate products like white bread and rice, soda, and highly processed baked goods. Does this sound familiar? Our plant-based recommendations, which are in no way low-carb, suggest making the same changes! Refined sugar and refined grains contain calories but have very little, if any, other nutritional value. These are known as empty calories. As you probably have experienced, it is very easy to eat too much of these foods.

These processed foods are significantly different than the whole foods we recommend throughout this book. Whole grains, legumes, fruits, and starchy vegetables contain the carbohydrates you need for fuel, protein, vitamins, minerals, fiber, and phytochemicals to boot!

CARBOHYDRATE CONSIDERATIONS FOR ATHLETES

Carbohydrates can be stored in your muscles and liver in the form of glycogen, the body's preferred and first-used source of fuel. Because glycogen is your body's go-to source of energy, starting a workout with high glycogen stores can prolong your effort and delay the onset of fatigue. Elite athletes, for example, can perform many hours of activity on very little food because of their ability to store large amounts of glycogen—this is part of the reason some top marathoners can complete the 26.2-mile distance without taking in anything besides water!

The other stored energy source we can draw upon is body fat. Most simply, body fat is just stored energy. When we eat excess calories, regardless of their source, we store the energy for later use as body fat.

When we work out, we start by using glycogen and only small amounts of body fat. As the workout or race progresses and our glycogen stores become depleted, our bodies slowly transition to using body fat for energy. But body

(continued)

fat isn't a quick source because it's not in a form immediately available for your muscles to use. Hence the need to continue the consumption of carbohydrate calories while working out or racing.

And like glycogen storage, we can improve our body's ability to burn fat as fuel. The more we work out and get into glycogen-depleted states, the better we can "switch" to using body fat as energy. But even the best-trained athletes can "bonk" or "hit the wall," which are phrases that describe glycogen storage depletion.

Athletes can increase their glycogen storage significantly by eating carbohydrate-rich meals soon after working out. This refueling will help you recover quicker, feel less fatigued from your workout, and prepare you better for your next workout. Although the science isn't entirely clear on this subject just yet, it is helpful to eat a small meal or snack within forty-five minutes after finishing your workout. Ideally, this meal should have a carbohydrate to protein ratio of 4:1 (for example, if your post-workout meal contains forty grams of carbohydrates, shoot for ten grams of protein).

Fiber–You Can Have Too Much of a Good Thing

For most people, making the transition to plant-based foods from the standard American diet involves seriously increasing the grams of fiber consumed per day. One benefit of fiber is that it promotes the movement of material through your digestive tract. In other words, increased bathroom breaks. Your body will adjust better to an increase in fiber when you add it slowly.

Also, some athletes report problems with fiber, such as stomach distress and increased bowel movements during exercise. If this is the case, reduce your fiber intake leading up to and during a competitive event or long training day. As a result, you might need to eat some extra refined carbohydrate to meet your caloric needs, and that's okay.

Any adjustment should be based on a balance of what your own body prefers and what you are comfortable eating. If most days your diet is very healthy, consisting of fruits, vegetables, and whole grains, then a few days eating lower-fiber foods will not affect your overall health. Some athletes look forward to these days to eat special foods they normally avoid, while others do not have to make any changes at all.

RECOMMENDED CARBOHYDRATE SOURCES

Complex carbohydrates:

- Brown rice
- Sweet potatoes
- Butternut and kabocha squash
- Whole-grain pastas, cereals, and breads
- Quinoa, oats, barley, millet, spelt, buckwheat, and other whole grains and pseudograins
- Beans and lentils

Simple carbohydrates:

- Fruit of all kinds

Protein: Building Muscles with Plant Foods

Oh, protein. It's the topic many amateur athletes think they are experts in, and one of the first targets of criticism in any discussion involving plant-based diets and sports. Many people believe a plant-based diet doesn't provide enough protein, but this isn't true. Protein is easy enough to obtain without eating meat. Let's start with understanding the science behind protein.

When we talk about protein, what we are really discussing are amino acids. These amino acids have specific roles in metabolism, muscle development, and wound healing. Nine of them can't be created by our bodies or from other amino acids and are therefore called "essential" amino acids.

When you hear about one protein source being better than another, it's in reference to the amino acid makeup. Some animal foods contain all of the amino acids in the amounts we need. If you ate only eggs and nothing else for months and months, for example, you would not develop an amino acid deficiency (but probably a host of other deficiencies!). Do the same with only lentils, however, and you may not get enough of the amino acid methionine.

Fortunately, no one eats like this. When we eat a variety of foods, most of which have some protein, at the end of the day we get all of the amino acids we need. The measure by which animal and vegetable proteins are usually compared is inadequate and outdated.

If you're eating enough for your activity level and consuming a variety of whole foods, you will get all the protein you need. For example, lentils and soymilk are made up of more than 30 percent protein. Even some foods we usually think of as purely carbohydrate sources contain a fair amount of protein—15 percent of the calories in whole wheat pasta are from protein, and even brown rice is about 8 percent protein.

How Much Protein Do You Need?

Between 10 and 20 percent of your total daily calories need to come from protein. High-protein foods include beans, nuts, seeds, and whole grains.

There are a few different ways to make protein recommendations. One is by grams based on your body weight. The Dietary Reference Intake (DRI), for example, recommends consuming 0.36 grams of protein per pound of body weight (or 0.8 grams per kilogram of body weight). This is useful for calculating out the number of grams of protein you need for each day. For example, if I weigh 175 pounds and need 0.36 grams of protein per pound of body weight, my daily protein need is sixty-three grams.

Another way to calculate protein requirements is as a percentage of the calories you eat each day, aiming for 10 to 20 percent of your total calories to come from protein. For example, if the calculations in the "Calculating Your Daily Calories" box on page 67 tell you that you need 2,400 calories per day to meet your protein needs, then you should shoot to get 240 to 480 of those calories from protein. Every gram of protein is four calories (each gram of carbohydrate is also four calories; a gram of fat is nine calories), so this equates to between 60 and 120 grams of protein each day. This range, of course, will vary depending on your particular daily total caloric needs.

Why the Advice That Athletes Need More Protein Is Misleading

Sure, athletes need more protein than non-athletes. But we also need more carbohydrates and fat. In fact, our overall caloric needs are much higher because we burn so much energy in our training.

Because we're eating more calories, we're automatically consuming more protein if we stay at 10 to 20 percent of our total. Let that sink in for a minute: as your caloric needs increase from the exercise you are doing, your intake of protein increases as well.

For example, I weigh about 175 pounds, and I need 2,500 calories most days. If I'm striving for 10 percent, then 250 of those calories need to be from protein. Dividing by four (the number of calories per gram of protein), this amounts to about sixty-three grams of protein as my recommended daily intake.

IS SOY SAFE?

Tofu and soybeans have been a part of people's diets for hundreds of years. Soy is a nutrient-dense bean with lots of protein, healthy plant fat, phytochemicals, and micronutrients. It's also a highly researched food. There are decades of studies showing that it is safe and that eating it reduces your LDL—your so-called "bad" cholesterol—and may lower your risk of cancer. There's even a Food and Drug Administration (FDA) statement on its ability to lower cholesterol. It takes hundreds of research articles and many years of evidence for the FDA to make such official statements. There are very few foods that have gone through such extensive scrutiny, and the evidence showing soybeans are healthy is strong.

After a food becomes extremely popular, two things usually happen: 1) Companies attempt to exploit the good research and add the food, or components of it, to existing products, and 2) there's a backlash when companies start adding the "miracle" food to other foods where it doesn't belong. (We don't need to add soybeans to potato chips—we should just eat the soybeans!) Both have happened with soy.

Here's what you need to know: Soybeans contain the beneficial phytochemical isoflavone. Isoflavones are plant estrogens, also known as phytoestrogens, but these are not the same as the hormone estrogen found in the human body, despite what some people think. Eating soy doesn't feminize men, affect sperm count, cause cancer, or negatively affect thyroid or cognitive function. It can and should be a part of a healthy diet, as long as that diet has variety! The best forms are the more whole-food options like tofu, tempeh, and edamame. Veggie burgers and "fake meat" products can be eaten regularly, just limit the very refined soy protein isolate. It's always best to eat the more whole-food version! For vegetarians and vegans it's easy to rely on soy products, but add other beans to your meals regularly and use soy products as a component of healthy diet, just not the only component.

For more information on soy, see two articles by Ginny Messina, M.P.H., R.D.: "Safety of Soyfoods" (www.vegetariannutrition.net/docs/Soy-Safety.pdf) and "Isoflavones" (www.vegetariannutrition.net/docs/Isoflavones-Vegetarian-Nutrition.pdf). Also see "Finally, the Truth About Soy", by Leo Babauta (www.zenhabits.net/soy).

When I'm training hard, I need more energy to fuel my longer, tougher workouts, and my total caloric needs can easily double (see how to calculate your daily caloric needs on page 67). Therefore, in order to maintain the proper protein/calorie ratio, so does my protein consumption.

Because athletes burn more calories than sedentary people and therefore require more calories, I tell the vegan athletes I consult to shoot for 0.45 to 0.55 grams of protein per pound of bodyweight (1.0 to 1.2 grams of protein per kilogram of body weight).

There's No Such Thing as an Incomplete Protein

If I am going to rid the world of ignorance about plant proteins, I'm going to start by eliminating the phrase "incomplete protein." It is misleading and biased and we should stop using it. When people say a protein is "incomplete," they are implying it is completely devoid of some amino acids. But here's the catch—all sources of protein have all of the essential amino acids! Some plant foods just don't have them all in the right amount if you were to only eat that one food forever.

The problem with the idea of complete and incomplete proteins is simple: *It assumes we only eat one type of food!* It's an example of a common mistake in nutrition: focusing on the specific nutrients of one food without seeing them in the context of an entire diet. Saying a protein is incomplete ignores the big picture and is often used as a critique of plant-based diets.

Although it's tempting to want to combine these "incomplete" proteins to form a whole, the truth is there's no need to combine protein sources within a given meal. Really. I know you have heard this one over and over—even the college textbook I teach from says it's a must!—but trust me, *it is not necessary to form complete proteins within a single meal.* Our bodies pool the amino acids we need as we eat them over a twenty-four-hour period, and we use them as needed.

Some complete protein combinations happen naturally—think pinto beans with rice, chickpeas with couscous, or granola with soymilk. But this is not a requirement for us to get all of the indispensable amino acids. Combining proteins was popularized in the 1970s by the influential book *Diet for a Small Planet,* by Francis Moore Lappe. Although combining plant proteins has been deemed unnecessary for decades—Lappe even added a statement in later editions about there being no need to combine proteins—the idea still lives on.

PROTEIN CONSIDERATIONS FOR ATHLETES

Seitan (a.k.a. wheat gluten or wheat meat) is a delicious alternative to meat that has become common at vegetarian restaurants and grocery stores. Gluten is the isolated protein from the wheat plant; therefore, these fake meat products are very high in protein and popular among some plant-based athletes.

Unfortunately, the digestibility of gluten is very low, and as such, it is not recommended as a main source of protein. Often fake meats are a combination of soy and gluten, so it's best to read the ingredient list and know what exactly you are eating. In short, gluten is fine to eat and not problematic for most people, but be sure to vary your protein sources and keep the emphasis on whole foods.

In addition to seitan, protein powder is a popular choice for plant-based athletes. It's unfortunate because most people, even athletes, can get enough protein from their regular diet without supplementing. Yes, powdered supplements are convenient, and it's not that they're unhealthy, but just know that it's possible to get enough protein without them before you buy in.

Who may need supplements? Two main groups of athletes: strength athletes who incorporate very little endurance training and those athletes who are attempting to drop weight while still training excessively hard. Both types of athletes may be looking to increase their protein intake without increasing total calories, with the result that the math in this chapter wouldn't add up. Hence, an efficient source of protein (meaning a source that contains protein and little else) is necessary, and here's where protein powder can help.

If you're going to use protein powder, a blend of hemp, rice, and pea proteins offers a balanced amino acid profile and is probably the best choice for plant-based athletes.

RECOMMENDED PROTEIN SOURCES

- Tempeh
- Lentils, black beans, chickpeas, and other beans
- Tofu
- Whole-food veggie burgers
- Nuts and nut butters

Even some whole grains, pseudograins, and green vegetables have 15 percent or more of their calories coming from protein.

Fat: A Beneficial Component of a Plant-Based Diet

Dietary fat is an important part of a solid nutrition plan, from the omega-3 and omega-6 fatty acids required by our bodies to the heart-healthy monounsaturated fats that can lower our cholesterol levels. Whole foods, as we've learned, are more than single sources of nutrients, and most foods contain all three sources of calories: carbohydrate, protein, and fat.

Fat contains nine calories per gram, more than twice as much as carbohydrate and protein. These calories can add up fast, which is what led to the low-fat craze of the 1990s. For example, one tablespoon (15 ml) of olive oil has 120 calories. Now compare that to broccoli: it takes six cups (426 g) to reach 120 calories! One-hundred and twenty calories of broccoli is chock full of nutrients like calcium and phytochemicals like lutein, while olive oil, for example, is almost 100 percent fat with few other nutrients.

Is Saturated Fat Bad for You?

Some newer studies have called into question the link between saturated fat (found in many animal products, especially dairy, but also in some plant foods like coconut) and heart disease. But these new studies don't overturn decades of research that shows saturated fat does indeed raise cholesterol levels and increase risk of heart disease. The new evidence shows the importance of what you replace the saturated fat with. If it's highly refined carbohydrate, then there's little or no reduction in risk. But when saturated fats are replaced with plant-based fats, there is a definite reduction in risk.

Additionally, overall diet patterns are much more important than single nutrients or factors. Should you eliminate saturated fat? If you are eating lots of whole plant foods, getting plenty of exercise, and don't smoke, my suggestion is to be mindful of saturated fats and limit them to less than 10 percent of total calories.

COCONUT: HEALTH FOOD OR FAD?

Coconut has gained significant popularity recently in the plant-based crowd, but is it a health food? The potential problem with coconut is its huge amount of saturated fat. Saturated fat intake is directly correlated with high cholesterol and the accompanying risk of heart disease.

What makes coconut unique is that it contains medium-chain triglycerides, which do not negatively impact your cholesterol levels. So this much is true: some of the saturated fat in coconut is not actually bad for you. But coconut fat (like lard) is high in myristic and palmitic acids, which do raise cholesterol levels.

Where does that leave us? Many years ago, when saturated fat was first implicated as a risk factor for high cholesterol, the food industry replaced it in common foods with processed, hydrogenated fat, a.k.a. trans-fatty acids. It didn't take long for the research to show that these trans-fats were bad for us and should be avoided. Now what?

It's always a better choice to eat whole foods than processed ones, even if they contain high amounts of fat. This way, the fat is part of a "nutrition package" and comes with other nutrients and beneficial components beyond just fat. While the jury is still out, there is some evidence that, despite containing large amounts of myristic and palmitic fatty acids, coconut consumption does not increase your risk for heart disease.

My opinion is that fat is part of a healthy diet, but you do need to keep in mind how much you eat and be conscious of your overall saturated fat consumption.

FUELING FOR THE "FASTEST GAME ON EARTH" WITH PLANTS

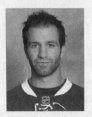

By Mike Zigomanis

National Hockey League (NHL) and American Hockey League (AHL) professional hockey player

I made the choice to eat a plant-based diet to improve my body's recovery time after training and injury, increase my energy and stamina, and improve my overall health and well-being.

I continue to eat a plant-based diet not only for my health, but for the health of the planet and its animals.

Once my body adjusted to the plant-based diet, I noticed an increase in energy, a quicker recovery time after training and injury, and an improvement in my quality of sleep. I feel just as strong, if not stronger, on the ice as I did before I switched to a plant-based diet.

I recommend that anyone making the switch from a traditional diet to take it slow. Listen to your body and make changes gradually.

I love to drink fresh juices and smoothies. They are a great way to pack in a lot of nutrients and protein on the go. Before I start a game, I take Vega Pre-Workout Energizer to increase my energy levels and sustain the endurance I need for battle. One of my favorite smoothies is made with Vega Sport Performance Protein Chocolate, almond butter, banana, water, and unsweetened almond milk.

Oil: Friend or Foe?

Certain advocates within the plant-based diet movement say that oil should be avoided because it's not a whole food. They are certainly correct that it's not a whole food, and there's no doubt that eating an olive is inherently more nutritious than just eating the oil that has been extracted from it—it'd take a lot of olives to get as many calories as you do in just a few tablespoons of oil.

As we've learned, some fat is beneficial. Olive oil, for instance, has a very good profile because it's high in monounsaturated fats, but it's still only one component of the bigger health picture. With that said, I do not think we need to avoid all oils. Oil plays several key roles that aren't directly related to its nutrition profile: it's required for the absorption of the fat-soluble vitamins A, D, E, and K, it may help with joint health, and it is a concentrated source of energy that can help athletes meet their high caloric needs. It's also beneficial in preparation and cooking because it can improve the texture and palatability of food and function as a flavor-carrier (it's why we add garlic and onions when we sauté foods).

Ultimately, it's up to you to decide whether oil has a place in your particular diet. Almost all of the recipes in this book can be modified to create oil-free versions, and guidelines are given at the beginning of chapter 6 to do so.

If you decide to use oil in your cooking, it's important to do the following:

▶ Use high-quality, expeller-pressed oil, instead of generic corn or soy vegetable oil that may be genetically modified (GM) and contain only small amounts of omega-3 or monounsaturated fats.

▶ When using oil to sauté vegetables, first heat the pan and then add the oil. When added to a hot pan, oil expands, allowing you to cover the pan in a thin layer of oil without using a lot of it.

▶ Consider whole food alternatives for recipes. Olives and nut butters are whole foods that can be blended to make sauces or dressings. In addition to the benefits from their quality fat content, these foods provide more micronutrients than the oil alone.

FAT CONSIDERATIONS FOR ATHLETES

Fat can be used to meet your overall caloric needs because it is more than twice as calorically dense as carbohydrate and protein. Before workouts, however, excess amounts of fat are not recommended as the pathway to turn fat to energy is slow.

Omega-3s: Get the Healthy Fish Fat without the Fish

Omega-3 fatty acids are nutritive—our bodies require them for growth and metabolism. The reason most people know about omega-3s is because this is the type of fat found in fish that is also associated with lower cholesterol levels. Fortunately, there are plant-based omega-3 sources, including flaxseeds, walnuts, hemp seeds, kale, and other leafy greens. That's right—leafy greens have some fat, and it's the good kind! Kale is about 12 percent fat, a significant amount of which is omega-3 fatty acids. The reason leafy greens are not commonly recommended as sources of fat is because they are so low in calories. One cup (67 g) of raw kale has only thirty-three calories and a half gram of fat. Put another way, you would have to eat two uncooked cups (134 g) of kale just to get one gram of fat!

There are a few technicalities regarding omega-3s that make recommendations difficult. Some evidence says that what's most important is your ratio of omega-6s to omega-3s. The ratio in the standard American diet is about 10:1, which is considered too high. There's no consensus yet on the ideal ratio, but it is definitely lower than 10:1. Oils like soybean and corn oil are high in omega-6s and low in omega-3s and therefore skew your fatty acid balance in the wrong direction. In the United States, most people have a less-than-ideal ratio because of the overconsumption of refined oils—more evidence that a whole foods diet is best!

To make sure you're getting a healthy amount of omega-3s, be sure to regularly consume flaxseeds, hemp seeds, or walnuts and don't hesitate to eat big portions of leafy greens like kale.

RECOMMENDED FAT SOURCES

- Walnuts and other nuts
- Nut butters
- Flax and other seeds
- Avocados
- Extra virgin olive oil and other oils, such as grapeseed, hemp, and coconut, all in moderation

Don't Forget These Other Necessary Nutrients

For your diet to be nutritionally adequate, you need to eat enough calories, as discussed previously, and also get all of the nutrients your body needs. By definition, nutrients are substances that provide nourishment essential for growth and the maintenance of life. In addition to the essential amino acids, fatty acids, and carbohydrates we've discussed so far, nutrients include vitamins and minerals. Each vitamin and mineral has very specific functions at the cellular level. Consider the additional nutrients below.

Vitamin B_{12}: Find This Essential Nutrient in Fortified Foods

If you are eating a plant-based diet, you need to know about vitamin B_{12} because it is crucial for our brains and nervous systems, red blood cells, and a host of other functions. Long-time deficiency can have irreversible health implications, including blindness and dementia. It's no joke! And you cannot get B_{12} from plant foods. It's not in tempeh, seaweed, or spirulina, despite what some individuals say.

Fortunately, B_{12} is available in prepared vegan foods, like fortified non-dairy milks, cereals, nutritional yeast, meat alternatives, and energy bars. Check the label though, because not all prepared fortified vegan foods are fortified with B_{12}. If you are not consuming a source of B_{12} every day, take a supplement or make sure your multivitamin contains B_{12}. Symptoms of deficiency include fatigue, numbness, nausea, impaired memory, and even depression. The recommended daily intake for healthy adults is 2.4 micrograms. This is a very small amount, but nonetheless crucial. For more information on B_{12}, I recommend reading the article "B_{12}: Are You Getting It?" (www.veganhealth. org/articles/vitaminb12) by Jack Norris, R.D.

Iron: Eat a Varied Diet to Avoid Deficiency

Iron deficiency is the most common nutrient deficiency in North America, with symptoms including fatigue, pale skin, weakness, and inability to maintain body temperature. And as vegetarians and vegans, it's worth paying special attention to make sure we're getting enough. How much iron do we actually need?

In 2001, the Institute of Medicine revised its Dietary Reference Intake (DRI) for iron, specifically for vegetarians—making it 1.8 times higher than for the general population. As my colleague Jack Norris points out, this increase is not based on research on vegetarians, but simply because the iron in plant foods is not as easily absorbed as the iron in animal products (more on this in just a minute). Many experts in vegetarian nutrition believe that these recommendations are much higher than needed.

My take on it: if you eat a varied, healthy, plant-based diet that includes a balance of grains, legumes, nuts, seeds, fruits, and vegetables and follow the recommendations in this section, you can get all the iron you need from plant foods.

EATING ENOUGH THROUGHOUT THE DAY

When you are physically active and eating mostly plant foods, some of the general rules about nutrition go out the window.

- **It's okay to snack.** Getting enough calories on plant foods to support your fitness training may require snacking throughout the day. Don't hesitate to eat when you are hungry! Snacking also helps prevent overeating during meal time.

- **There's also nothing wrong with eating at night.** It's a long-standing myth that you shouldn't eat at night. Although it's probably best not to eat a meal and go to sleep for the night immediately after (mainly because this could diminish the quality of your sleep), eating late is not a problem, especially when you need the calories to replenish what you expended during the day and for storage for your next day's workouts.

Iron from Plants vs. Iron from Animals

To better understand what we need to do to ensure our bodies are getting enough iron, we first have to accept two facts about iron, painful as they may be for vegetarians and vegans to hear:

1. There are two types of iron: heme, which is found in animal foods, and non-heme, which is from plants. Heme iron is better absorbed than non-heme iron.

2. Vegetarians and vegans may have lower iron stores than omnivores.

But don't fret! We'll see that, in fact, it's not all that difficult to get the iron you need on a plant-based diet. As for the second fact, though vegetarians have lower stores of iron than omnivores, they do not have higher rates of anemia. According the review of research done for *The Academy of Nutrition and Dietetics Position Paper on Vegetarian Diets* in 2009, many vegetarians' stores are "low-normal," but this does not mean less than ideal! Actually, there's some evidence that says low-normal iron stores are beneficial because they can improve insulin function and lower rates of heart disease and cancer.

It's not how much iron you consume, but how well you absorb it.

To get enough iron on a plant-based diet, start by eating foods that contain substantial amounts of iron. Some of the best plant sources of iron include the following:

▶ Legumes: lentils, soybeans, tofu, tempeh, lima beans, and peanuts

▶ Grains and pseudograins: quinoa, fortified cereals, brown rice, and oatmeal

▶ Nuts and seeds: pumpkin, squash, pine, pistachio, sunflower, cashews, and unhulled sesame

▶ Vegetables: tomato sauce, Swiss chard, and collard greens

▶ Other: blackstrap molasses, and prune juice

But here's the key: It's not how much iron you consume, but how well you absorb it. Fortunately, there are four great ways to increase the absorption of non-heme iron:

1. The less iron you take in at a time, the better it is absorbed. When consuming larger amounts of iron at one time, the percentage that our bodies absorb is actually lower than when your meal contains only a few milligrams. Eating smaller amounts throughout the day is a great way to increase absorption.

2. Eat non-heme iron foods with vitamin C foods, and absorption can increase as much as five times. Five times! Culturally, these combinations are already happening: think beans and rice with salsa, falafel with tomatoes, and hummus with lemon juice. The iron in beans, grains, and seeds is better absorbed when combined with the vitamin C found in fruits and vegetables. Bonus: some iron sources, such as leafy greens, broccoli, and tomato sauce, already contain vitamin C.

3. Avoid coffee and tea when eating high-iron meals. Coffee, even decaffeinated, and tea contain tannins that inhibit iron absorption. I recommend avoiding them an hour before or two hours after your meal.

4. Cast-iron skillets increase iron absorption. Cooking with an old school cast-iron skillet increases the iron in your meal, especially when you cook food containing vitamin C in the skillet. Even better, a cast-iron skillet purchase puts you in the realm of official serious cook. I bought mine almost ten years ago for $8, and it is one of my most valued possessions.

Eating good sources of iron throughout the day using these absorption principles will make it easy to get enough iron in your diet as a plant-based athlete.

All of that said, iron is one of the few nutrients where a deficiency both immediately affects your health and is detectable, so if you have any iron-deficiency symptoms, I recommend getting blood work with your doctor—it is affordable, reliable, and easy to interpret. And iron levels bounce back quickly when using the methods above or taking a supplement.

IRON CONSIDERATIONS FOR ATHLETES

In addition to its role in helping hemoglobin carry oxygen to your cells, iron is found in myoglobin in your muscles and involved in making amino acids. Therefore, getting enough iron is especially important for athletes and even more so during periods of heavy training. Use the tips in this section to make sure you are getting enough iron and that it is getting absorbed. If you are eating packaged energy bars or other snacks, look closely at the label to make sure they contain iron.

Phytonutrients, Phytochemicals, and Antioxidants

Phyto (meaning plant) nutrients, often referred to as phytochemicals, are chemicals found in many plant foods that are believed to confer protective effects on health. They are different from vitamins and minerals in that they are not essential nutrients, like amino acids and carbohydrates (for example) are. There are literally thousands of phytochemicals that have been identified! Often foods with high amounts of phytonutrients are labeled as superfoods.

Phytonutrients are found in almost all plant foods, including fruits, vegetables, grains, legumes, nuts, seeds, spices, herbs, and cacao, as well as in beverages like tea and coffee. Many act as antioxidants and protect the body from free radical damage to cell membranes, DNA molecules, and other important areas and processes in the body. When oxygen interacts with cells of any type, damage can occur—like an apple that browns after being cut. The same damage, called free radical damage, can occur to our cells. Antioxidants that we eat help reduce the overall damage that is done by this oxidation.

Studies have reported that vegetarians have higher intakes of antioxidants and phytochemicals and greater plasma antioxidant levels than omnivores.

For athletes, consumption of phytochemicals may aid in recovery and reduce overall recovery time. Plant-based diets contain high levels of phytonutrients because all whole foods contain phytonutrients. Studies looking at differences between omnivores and vegetarians have reported that vegetarians have higher intakes of antioxidants and phytochemicals and greater plasma antioxidant levels than omnivores, which may partly explain the lower incidence of some chronic diseases in vegetarians and vegans.

Phytonutrient research is the future of nutrition and one can only hypothesize that as we learn more about these extraordinary compounds, the benefits of plant-based diets will continue to be proven.

BOOST YOUR MICRONUTRIENT INTAKE: GET STARTED WITH RAW FOODS

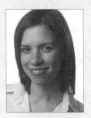

By Gena Hamshaw, C.C.N.
Certified clinical nutritionist, VegNews contributor, and blogger at Choosing Raw (www.choosingraw.com)

If you spend any time in the nutrition and wellness world, chances are you've heard of the raw food diet. Traditionally, raw foodism has been envisioned as a way of eating that seeks to preserve enzymes in food. Enzymes, which are proteins, are involved in the activation of biochemical reactions. Most of the enzymes used in the human body are denatured—or rendered inactive—at temperatures higher than 115°F (46° C).

The food we eat is rich in enzymes, but our bodies also produce digestive enzymes to break it down. One of the major tenets of the raw food philosophy is that if you preserve enzymes in food by never heating it above 115°F (46°C), those enzymes will go on to participate in food digestion. Your body will need to produce fewer enzymes of its own, and the energy it might spend on enzyme production and digestion can be directed elsewhere—to healing, assisting all metabolic processes, and building strong immunity.

Sounds pretty intuitive, right? Unfortunately, the science behind enzyme theory is murky at best and lacking at worst. Enzyme theory fails to account for the fact that enzymes are denatured by the heavily acidic environment of the stomach (a pH of about 3). They'll then be broken down into amino acids and digested like any protein would be. Ultimately, the body's digestive enzymes will be called upon to aid in this digestive process, whether you've heated your food or not. Some vegan health practitioners claim that certain enzymes may survive the digestion process, but if this is true, it is likely to be only a small amount.

NO MEAT
ATHLETE

If the central tenet of raw foodism is not supported by science, then why eat raw? As it turns out, there are tons of reasons. Part of it is aesthetic. I love the simplicity, color, and freshness of raw cuisine. When I first discovered raw foods, I had been on a steady diet of rice, beans, tofu, and cooked veggies. I was bored and uninspired. Raw foods presented me with bright hues, crunchy textures, and endless culinary creativity. It takes a lot of imagination to create satisfying cuisine without cooking; not surprisingly, raw food chefs are known for their innovation.

Although enzyme preservation may not be so ultimately important, there is good evidence to show that eating foods raw can preserve some of their vital micronutrients (minerals and vitamins). Vitamin C, in particular, is susceptible to diminishment through cooking. So are certain phytochemicals—the plant compounds that may be so helpful in fighting cancer and free radical damage. And mineral loss from cooking has been estimated in some studies to be as high as 30 to 40 percent. It's important to note that not all foods are best eaten raw; the cancer-fighting compound lycopene, for instance, is released when tomatoes are cooked.

But variety is important. Before I began eating raw food, it was easy for me to cook virtually all of my vegetables except for my salads. Today, I'm mindful to create raw slaws, marinated vegetables, and other dishes with raw and cooked ingredients. As a result, my diet has become more nutrient dense, more variable, and a lot more interesting.

The final reason raw foods appeal to me is more complex than aesthetics, taste, or nutrition. Raw foods force us to be involved with our food preparation, to pay attention to the quality and integrity of our ingredients. They encourage us to showcase food in its natural state; they are the earth's raw materials (pun intended).

There's no one right or wrong way to get started with raw food. You can begin by adding a green smoothie to your morning routine. You can swap a standard lunch wrap or sandwich with a big salad, packed with nuts, seeds, avocado, and some sprouted or cooked legumes. You can make a batch of cashew cheese and layer it between zucchini, tomato, and basil slices for a quick and easy raw lasagna. A lot of people find that raw entrées such as this

(continued)

may not be filling enough on their own. To make your raw dish heartier, serve it with cooked legumes, cooked root veggies, or quinoa. Remember, the goal is not to be exclusively raw, so it doesn't matter if you mix raw and cooked foods in the same meal. In fact, because variety is so beneficial, a mixture of raw and cooked foods is ideal. My favorite high-raw dishes include the following:

Breakfast:

- Green smoothie
- Raw fruit/nut bar and salad
- Sprouted lentils, vegetables, and avocado
- Banana wrapped in romaine lettuce with almond butter
- Chia seed pudding

Lunch:

- Large salad, packed with fat and protein
- Raw nori sushi rolls with a nut "paté" filling
- "Rice" made from jicama or cauliflower, tossed with mixed veggies and some lentils or (cooked) chickpeas
- Sprouted grain bread (I like Ezekiel or Manna bread) with avocado and a salad
- Raw soup and salad

Dinner:

- Raw parsnip rice with cooked butternut squash and creamy cashew sauce
- Zucchini "spaghetti" with raw tomato sauce and lentils
- Raw marinated portobello mushrooms with raw "mashed potatoes" (made from cauliflower and cashews!)

See? It's not quite as exotic as it may sound. If you pick the right recipes, raw foodism can be easy, fun, and stress free. As a full time pre-medical student and blogger, I have relied on "uncooking" to fuel my hectic lifestyle. Just play around with a few raw recipes, paying close attention to the beauty of your food as you go along. I hope you'll be as inspired and excited about this brave new world of food preparation as I always have been.

CHAPTER 4

IN THE KITCHEN: BASIC COOKING SKILLS TO SAVE YOU TIME, ENERGY, AND EMBARRASSMENT

Okay, you're on board with the plant-based diet! Now what's the first step to becoming healthier than ever? The simplest answer is this: Start cooking. Michael Pollan, author of *In Defense of Food* and a fellow advocate of getting into the kitchen as the way to eating healthier, sums it up well when he points out that nobody reaches for the bottle of high-fructose corn syrup when they're in their own kitchen.

Whether plant-based or still omnivorous, your diet will improve the day you start cooking because it forces you to become aware of every ingredient you put into your food and your body. Especially for plant-based eaters, for whom healthy and substantial restaurant choices are often few and far between, cooking your own food isn't an option, it's a must.

Many people are afraid of cooking. It overwhelms and intimidates them, and they assume cooking is some magical skill that you either have or you don't. But the fear is really unfounded. Cooking is an easy skill to learn, and it's quite rewarding when you combine a few humble ingredients and produce something delicious, comforting, and nourishing. Cooking is also one of the most valuable skills you can acquire, as cooking your own food will save you a tremendous amount of money over the long haul, not to mention make whomever you live with very happy.

How to Start Cooking Today

Here's the secret to cooking for those who have never tried: If you can follow directions, you can cook. Recipes make it incredibly easy to get in the kitchen and start cooking. Most of them assume no knowledge or cooking ability, and thanks to the Internet, many of them are now available for free. This is pretty incredible—you and I can cook dishes at home that the best chefs in the world spent hours of time and energy developing and at no cost other than the price of the food itself.

In this book, I've included my favorite plant-based recipes that aren't just healthy, but substantial enough for athletes. Several of the recipes are also designed specifically for sports—high-carbohydrate meals for loading up before an endurance event or long workout, energy drinks and gels to keep you going strong, and post-workout recovery smoothies and meals to jumpstart the process of repairing your muscles so you can get back out there soon to do it all again.

In addition to the requirement that the recipes be both delicious and suitable for athletes, I made them as simple as possible. I love cooking and often spend several hours making dinner on the weekend, but I recognize that most athletes would much rather be outside training than stuck in the kitchen.

The recipes are simple enough that you should be able to execute all of them with little or no cooking experience. But the experience will become far more pleasurable as you develop a basic familiarity with common cooking techniques, learn a few time-saving tricks, and avoid potential pitfalls.

To help you move more quickly through the learning curve, in this short chapter I'll highlight the most valuable skills I picked up in my first few years of cooking, which you should be able to apply immediately to your cooking and save yourself all (okay, most) of the mistakes I made.

The Four Most Important Kitchen Time-Savers

If you just want to get your hands dirty and start cooking, by all means feel free to make some of the recipes before you've read this entire section. But the information here will ultimately save you tons of time and mistakes, and taking a few minutes to read and understand it is an investment that will pay dividends immediately.

1. Chop and prepare your ingredients before you start cooking.

Trying to keep up with a recipe can be a little stressful at first, and one of the easiest ways to stay on top of things is to handle all your prep in advance. (This is known as *mise en place*, which is French for "everything in place.")

Once you're comfortable in the kitchen and faster with chopping, and especially once you've made a recipe a couple times and you know what to expect, you can do much of your prep while certain ingredients cook to speed things up. But at first, having everything in place before you dive in will save you immeasurable stress and prevent many burned dishes and ruined meals.

2. Keep a garbage bowl nearby as you prep.

This is one of the simplest things you can do to speed up the preparation process. It requires almost no explanation: instead of many trips across the kitchen to the garbage can, opening and closing the lid each time, you just toss your scraps into a bowl and empty it into the trash or compost heap once the meal is finished. It doesn't seem like much, but the five or ten trips to the trash can add up as you prep a meal, and it's much easier to get into the flow of cooking without them.

3. Invest in one or two quality knives, keep them honed and sharpened, and learn to use them.

You've probably heard that you're more likely to cut yourself with a dull knife than a sharp one. The reason is that you have to apply a lot of pressure to get a dull knife to cut, which leads to slips. If the knives you currently own haven't been cared for (or are cheapos), you'll probably want to get some new ones.

I've found that a single, large (8- or 9-inch [20 to 23 cm]) chef's knife and a small paring knife are all that I need. There are a few occasions where a mid-sized utility knife comes in handy, but it's certainly not essential for a home cook.

Your new knives will be very sharp at first, and you'll wonder how you ever got by with anything else. But that sharp edge won't last forever, so for any knife you're using regularly, I'd recommend having it sharpened by a professional every few months, and that assumes you keep it honed with a sharpening steel before each use.

You should get a sharpening or knife steel (that long, thin rod that comes with a knife set that almost nobody uses) to keep your knives honed between sharpenings. Although it doesn't technically "sharpen" the knife by removing metal from the blade, it lines up the molecules to produce a thinner edge. Get in the habit of running your knife along your steel a few times in each direction before every use, as demonstrated at the following website: http://video.about.com/housewares/How-to-Use-a-Knife-Steel.htm.

As for knife skills, there are well-established methods for chopping specific ingredients, but a general chopping principle is to first cut thin strips, then line up those strips and make uniform crosswise cuts from them. Think of carrots and celery, to which most people do the complete opposite by making crosswise cuts first, and then chopping over the whole pile of cross-sections. Instead, you want to cut even strips first, then run down the pile of strips once to get uniform dice in the fewest amount of cuts.

There are a few simple safeguarding techniques, such as hand position, you can use to prevent the major injuries that are possible in the kitchen, but it will be far easier for you to learn these methods visually than it would be to try to decipher them from text in a book. There's a thorough series of video- and photo-aided tutorials on basic knife skills, including knife safety, at the following website: http://culinaryarts.about.com/od/knifeskills/tp/knifeskills.htm.

4. Learn to quickly estimate amounts of ingredients.

Bill Buford, in his book *Heat*, says it best (you'll have to excuse the glaring non-veganism of the following excerpt, or replace the dirty words with "tofu"):

> Do you really believe the *Babbo* cookbook when it tells you that a linguine with eels takes four garlic cloves, that a lobster spaghettini takes two, and that the chitarra takes three? No. It's the same for each: a small pinch.

Meticulous measurement is one of the biggest time-killers in the kitchen, so unless you're baking, when exact measurements are crucial, stop measuring! Really, just stop. Those round numbers in recipes are just estimates anyway, and you'll learn a lot about flavors and gain some confidence by making a few mistakes in your own estimates.

For example, instead of measuring out a teaspoon of a spice each time a recipe calls for one, learn just once what a teaspoon of ground spice looks like in your hand or how many cranks of your pepper grinder it takes to grind a teaspoon of black pepper.

For oil, a good rule of thumb is that one drizzle around the pan is equal to about a tablespoon (15 ml), but it's instructive to actually measure out a tablespoon (15 ml) of oil and see what it looks like in the pan. Once you've done that, you can skip the measuring part—a tiny bit more or less oil isn't going to make a difference.

For solids, like nut butter, coconut oil, or anything semi-solid, 2 tablespoons (28 g) are about the same size as a ping-pong ball. You can find many more handy estimation tricks in my blog post at www.nomeatathlete.com/kitchen-time-savers.

Most Importantly: Get Started!

I can't overstress the importance and long-term positive impact on your health, and that of your family, of becoming comfortable in the kitchen. Don't let fear keep you from jumping in!

And just in case you're still apprehensive, rest assured, there are absolutely no cooking techniques in this book that a real chef would consider even remotely advanced. We're talking basic, cooking 101 stuff here. Anything else would miss the entire point of providing you with simple, healthy, delicious, plant-based recipes to support your training—I know you've got plenty of other places to spend your time and effort than in the kitchen.

Congratulations, You Know What It Takes. Have You Taken Action?

With that, we've reached the end of the nutrition section of this book, save for the recipes in the next chapter. What this means is that you're armed with all you need to make your plant-based diet work! In fact, you have more information than most new vegetarians and vegans have and far more than I knew when I decided to make the switch.

My hope is that by now you've already gotten started and taken the step that matters—the action. Reading and acquiring information is fantastic, but it doesn't mean a thing unless you put it to use. And for many people with all the best intentions, action will be the one step that doesn't happen.

Now is the time to start. There's no reason you need to finish Section 2, the running and fitness section of the book, before you can start your new, plant-based diet or your unique process of getting there—whether that means starting with just one plant-based day a week or going with the "fewer legs" approach described earlier. Choose a few recipes from the next chapter and use the tips in Chapter 2 to make this way of eating a habit, if you haven't yet.

And when you're ready—once you've started—I'll see you in Section 2: Running on Plants, where we'll dive into the fitness component of the No Meat Athlete lifestyle. See you there!

CHAPTER 5

RECIPES TO FUEL PLANT-BASED ATHLETES (AND THEIR FAMILIES, TOO!)

These recipes represent the No Meat Athlete nutritional philosophy in action. They are not only healthy and substantial enough to support active people, but also approachable, family-friendly, and most importantly, workable in the real world, even for those who are new to a plant-based diet. The following are a few notes to keep in mind regarding the use of oil and salt.

As Matt Ruscigno wrote in chapter 3, we consider certain oils to be healthy and beneficial in moderate amounts and when not heated above their smoke points. If you choose to limit oil intake more than we do, in almost all cases you can reduce the amount of oil called for in the recipes. Vegetable stock is often a decent substitute for oil, and it even works (in most cases) for sautéing. Sometimes, like in the hummus recipes in this chapter, the liquid from a can of beans that's called for in the recipe can stand in for oil as well. Substituting, reducing, or omitting the oils in the dessert recipes, however, is not recommended unless you know what you're doing.

As for salt, I consider a small amount of coarse, minimally processed, and mineral-rich sea salt to be a healthy, flavor-enhancing addition to most recipes, especially because so much sodium is cut from your diet when you stop eating packaged and fast foods. However, if for any reason you wish to use less salt than is called for in a recipe, you should be able to do so without a problem. One way to reduce salt intake is to only salt the finished meal, rather than adding it throughout the cooking process.

Substantial Soups and Salads

Smoothies, Energy Bars, and Food for Sports

Main-Event Meals

Super Sides, Snacks, and Sauces

Sneaky-Healthy Desserts

SUBSTANTIAL SOUPS AND SALADS

HEARTY CHICKPEA PASTA SOUP

Many authentic Italian dishes are based on the nutritious pairing of pasta and beans. Pasta e fagioli, which means "pasta and beans" in Italian, is a popular example, and this soup is my favorite spinoff of that classic, using chickpeas instead of the more traditional cannellini beans and rosemary as the standout flavor.

¼ cup (60 ml) extra virgin olive oil
1 small onion, chopped
2 celery ribs, diced
4 cloves garlic, minced
2 teaspoons fresh rosemary, finely chopped, divided
1 cup (245 g) any tomato sauce
6 cups (1.4 L) vegetable stock
1 can (15 ounces or 425 g) or 1½ cups (246 g) cooked chickpeas, drained and rinsed

1 bunch kale (about 8 leaves), preferably lacinato (also called dinosaur kale), torn into bite-size pieces, coarse stems removed
4 ounces (115 g) whole wheat or alternative-grain linguine, broken into 1 to 2 inch (2.5 to 5 cm) lengths (or choose a bite-size pasta)
1 teaspoon sea salt, or to taste
½ teaspoon fresh ground black pepper

Heat the oil in a large pot over medium heat. Add the onion, celery, garlic, and 1 teaspoon of the rosemary and cook until the vegetables are soft and translucent, about 5 minutes.

Add the tomato sauce, vegetable stock, and chickpeas, and bring to a boil. Add the kale and after about 5 minutes, add the pasta and stir occasionally. (This assumes your pasta will take 7 to 8 minutes to cook. If you're using pasta that takes 12 to 15 minutes, add the pasta when you add the kale.) When the pasta is al dente, remove the soup from the heat and season with salt and pepper.

Garnish with the remaining teaspoon of fresh rosemary and optionally, a drizzle of olive oil.

YIELD: ABOUT 6 SERVINGS

PER SERVING: 496 Calories; 20 g Fat (34.7% calories from fat); 16 g Protein; 67 g Carbohydrate; 9 g Dietary Fiber; 2 mg Cholesterol; 2140 mg Sodium

SENTIMENTAL LENTIL SOUP

Are lentils the perfect bean? They are high in protein, cook without being soaked, and easily turn into delicious soup! What makes this soup unique is the use of whole cumin seeds. The taste difference between the seed and the powder is indescribable, and you'll soon be nostalgic over this soup! —Matthew Ruscigno

2 tablespoons (28 ml) olive oil
2 teaspoons cumin seeds
1 small onion, chopped
4 cloves garlic, minced
1 teaspoon dried oregano
$\frac{1}{2}$ teaspoon red pepper flakes, more to taste
$\frac{1}{2}$ teaspoon salt

4 carrots, sliced
2 to 4 stalks celery, chopped
2 cups (384 g) dry brown lentils, picked over
8 cups (1.9 L) water or vegetable broth, warmed
Salt and black pepper, to taste
Juice of 1 lemon (optional)

Heat the olive oil in a large pot on medium heat. When hot, add the cumin seeds and toast for about one minute. As soon as they are fragrant, but before they turn black, add the onion. (This is the most difficult part of this recipe, but using whole cumin seeds is also the most rewarding.)

After a minute, add the garlic, oregano, red pepper flakes, and salt. When the garlic is fragrant, after about one minute, add the carrots and celery and sauté for 2 minutes. Add the lentils, stir, and heat for 2 minutes.

Add the water or broth (I like to preheat it so it gets up to temperature quicker), bring to a boil, and reduce heat to a simmer and cover. Cook for about 45 minutes or until lentils are soft.

Add salt and pepper to taste and lemon juice, if using. Enjoy! This soup makes for great leftovers, too.

YIELD: ABOUT 6 SERVINGS

PER SERVING: 292 Calories; 5 g Fat (16.1% calories from fat); 19 g Protein; 45 g Carbohydrate; 22 g Dietary Fiber; 0 mg Cholesterol; 224 mg Sodium

SOUTH-OF-THE-BORDER TORTILLA BLACK BEAN SOUP

Corn tortillas, especially if you make them at home or can get homemade ones at your local co-op, have an authentic flavor that wheat tortillas just can't match. This soup incorporates corn tortillas, which are eventually pureed, to add heartiness and flavor. To give the soup some extra heft, stir in 2 to 3 cups (390 to 585 g) of cooked brown rice near the end of the simmering time. If you're feeling extravagant, fry a few extra tortillas until they're very crispy and then chop them up to use for a garnish.

2 tablespoons (28 ml) grapeseed oil

4 corn tortillas (6 inches [15 cm]), roughly chopped

1 cup corn, fresh (154 g) or frozen (164 g) and thawed

4 cloves garlic, roughly chopped

1 small onion, roughly chopped

1 small jalapeño pepper, seeded, ribbed, and roughly chopped

1 tablespoon (7 g) ground cumin

2 cans (15 ounces, or 425 g) diced tomatoes

2 tablespoons (32 g) tomato paste

8 cups (1.9 L) vegetable stock

2 cans (15½ ounces, or 440 g) or 3 cups (516 g) cooked black beans, drained and rinsed

Salt and freshly ground black pepper, to taste

Juice of 1 lime plus more for serving

1 avocado, peeled, pitted, and diced, for garnish

Large handful fresh cilantro, chopped, for garnish

In a large soup pot, heat the oil over medium heat. Once the oil is hot, add the chopped tortillas and let them crisp up for two to three minutes.

Add the corn, garlic, onion, jalapeño, and cumin and stir to coat the vegetables. After 30 seconds, add the tomatoes and tomato paste. Stir to dissolve the tomato paste and add the vegetable stock. Increase the heat to bring the soup to a boil and then lower to medium, cover, and simmer for 30 minutes.

Being very careful not to scald yourself, use an immersion blender to puree the soup or transfer in batches to a food processor or regular blender to purée, venting regularly. Then add the black beans and allow them to heat through.

Season with salt and pepper, stir in lime juice, and serve garnished with avocado, cilantro, and additional lime juice to taste.

YIELD: 8 TO 10 SERVINGS

PER SERVING: 439 Calories; 12 g Fat (23.9% calories from fat); 17 g Protein; 69 g Carbohydrate; 13 g Dietary Fiber; 2 mg Cholesterol; 1478 mg Sodium

CHOPZILLA! SALAD

I haven't always loved salad. The truth is, I was vegan for a long time before I regularly made my own. What I learned is that I don't like other people's salads! That, and the key is to dice everything into small pieces—I don't want giant chunks of cucumbers in there! This salad needs to become your own. What I've written below is what works for me, but the magic is playing around with ingredients until you find your own Chopzilla!
—Matthew Ruscigno

1 pound (455 g) spring mix salad greens
2 bell peppers (red are my favorite)
1 cucumber, half peeled
1/2 head purple cabbage
1 zucchini
1 head broccoli
2 carrots

1/2 avocado, pitted and peeled
1/4 cup (30 g) toasted walnuts, chopped
1/4 cup (36 g) sunflower seeds
1 tablespoon (15 ml) flax oil
Juice of 1 lemon (optional)
1/4 cup (24 g) nutritional yeast
Salt and pepper, to taste

Chop all the veggies into small pieces (even the salad greens!). Add the remainder of the ingredients and mix well before serving.

YIELD: 4 SERVINGS OR 2 GIANT DINNER-SALAD SERVINGS

PER SERVING: 301 Calories; 14 g Fat (37.3% calories from fat); 19 g Protein; 36 g Carbohydrate; 17 g Dietary Fiber; 0 mg Cholesterol; 98 mg Sodium

SERVING SUGGESTIONS

The possibilities are endless here—don't be limited by conventional salads! Consider adding a cup of marinated tofu (240 g), black beans (172 g), or edamame (150 g) for additional protein and texture. For sweetness, add a quarter cup of raisins (35 g) or cranberries (30 g) or a diced apple (38 g). And sometimes the best ingredients are whatever happens to be on sale at your local grocery store or farmers market.

GODDESS DRESSING

I recently tasted goddess dressing for the first time (I've always been an oil-and-balsamic kinda guy) and my first reaction was, "Wow, I'd eat a lot more salads if I always had a bottle of this on hand!" This is my homemade version that's pretty darn close to what you can buy in the store. You can reduce the oil somewhat if you like.

¹/₄ cup (65 g) tahini
3 tablespoons (45 ml) apple
   cider vinegar
2 tablespoons (28 ml) tamari
1 tablespoon (15 ml) lemon juice
1 small clove garlic, minced

¹/₂ cup (120 ml) grapeseed oil
1 tablespoon (4 g) fresh parsley,
   finely chopped
1 tablespoon (6 g) scallions, finely
   chopped

In a medium bowl, whisk together all of the ingredients except the oil, parsley, and scallions. Slowly stream in the oil, whisking as you pour. When the oil is incorporated into the dressing, stir in the parsley and scallions.

YIELD: 1 CUP (235 ML)

TOTAL RECIPE: 1360 Calories; 141 g Fat (90.1% calories from fat); 14 g Protein; 20 g Carbohydrate; 6 g Dietary Fiber; 0 mg Cholesterol; 2084 mg Sodium

SERVING SUGGESTION

I like to use this Goddess dressing not just on salads, but as the sauce for tempeh "Caesar" salad pizza. Make the pizza crust (page 138) and top it after baking with sautéed or baked tempeh, romaine lettuce, and this dressing.

CO-OP TEMPEH SALAD

The French Broad Food Co-op near my house in Asheville, North Carolina, sells a prepared tempeh salad that's as good as any mayo-based salad I ate before I was vegan. My wife and I love it so much that we spent an afternoon trying to recreate it in our kitchen, and this is what we came up with. It's pretty close to the original!

FOR THE SALAD

8 ounces (225 g) tempeh, sliced into
   ½-inch (1.3 cm) blocks
2 celery stalks, diced
½ small onion, finely chopped
½ large or 1 small carrot, shredded
½ cup sundried tomatoes (avoid oil-
   packed), chopped
24 kalamata olives (about 1/2 cup [85 g]
   whole), pitted and chopped

FOR THE DRESSING

2 teaspoons Dijon mustard
3 tablespoons (42 g) vegan mayonnaise
   substitute
1 tablespoon (15 ml) plus 1 teaspoon
   apple cider vinegar
½ teaspoon sea salt
½ teaspoon fresh ground black pepper

To make the salad: Steam the tempeh for 20 minutes to remove any bitter taste and allow it to cool. When the tempeh is cool enough to handle, chop or crumble it into very small pieces.

In a large bowl, combine the tempeh, celery, onion, carrot, sundried tomatoes, and olives.

To make the dressing: In a small bowl, whisk together the dressing ingredients, pour over the salad ingredients, and stir to combine.

Serve by itself, over a green salad, or stuffed into a pita.

YIELD: 4 LUNCH-SIZE SERVINGS

PER SERVING: 255 Calories; 16 g Fat (52.5% calories from fat); 12 g Protein; 20 g Carbohydrate; 2 g Dietary Fiber; 0 mg Cholesterol; 816 mg Sodium

RECIPE VARIATION

This salad is so convenient for quick lunches, cookouts, and picnics that you'll want to mix it up now and then. For an easy curried variation, add 1 tablespoon (6.3 g) curry powder to the finished salad, more to taste, and stir to combine.

CHICKPEA AND CITRUS SALAD

Chickpea, garbanzo, ceci bean, chana, Gonzo Bean, Bengal gram—call them whatever you want. I call them delicious! This salad features a great balance of hearty beans, crisp greens, and bright citrus flavors. Note: If you're using freshly-sprouted chickpeas, skip the "For the chickpeas" section and simply add two cups (480 g) of sprouted chickpeas directly to the salad. If you are soaking dry chickpeas overnight, this recipe will make much more than two servings, so plan another chickpea meal this week. —Mo Ferris, Johnson & Wales–trained chef and vegetarian marathoner

FOR THE CHICKPEAS:

2 cups (400 g) dried chickpeas, soaked
   overnight or 6 to 8 hours
1/4 onion, rough chopped
1/2 celery stalk, rough chopped
1/2 carrot, peeled and rough chopped
1 bay leaf
2 teaspoons salt

FOR THE DRESSING:

1 tablespoon (15 ml) champagne vinegar
Juice of 1/2 lemon

1 teaspoon Dijon mustard
1/2 tablespoon agave nectar or maple
   syrup
Salt, to taste
Pinch fresh ground black pepper
1/3 cup (80 ml) extra virgin olive oil

FOR THE SALAD:

1 cup (75 g) Napa cabbage, very thinly
   sliced and chopped
1 tablespoon (4 g) fresh chopped parsley
Salt and pepper, to taste

To make the chickpeas: Place all the chickpea ingredients into a large, heavy-bottomed stockpot and cover with water. Bring to a boil, reduce heat to a low boil, and cook until chickpeas are tender, about 45 minutes. Drain. Discard onion, celery, carrot, and bay leaf. Spread chickpeas onto a sheet pan and cool completely.

To make the dressing: In a small food processor or blender, combine all the ingredients except the olive oil. Once blended and while the food processor or blender is running, gradually add olive oil to form an emulsion.

To make the salad: In a large mixing bowl, combine 2 cups (480 g) cooked or sprouted chickpeas, Napa cabbage, and parsley. Add vinaigrette and mix until all the ingredients are well coated. Season with salt and pepper.

YIELD: 2 SERVINGS

PER SERVING (excluding unknown items): 396 Calories; 22 g Fat (47.7% calories from fat); 12 g Protein; 41 g Carbohydrate; 11 g Dietary Fiber; 0 mg Cholesterol; 1685 mg Sodium

SUSAN'S MASSAGED KALE SALAD

When I'm ravenously hungry, I eat on one of two sides of the food spectrum: pizza delivery or kale. Thankfully, it's faster to make this kale salad than to wait for the pizza guy.
—Susan Lacke, No Meat Athlete*'s resident triathlete*

¹/₄ cup (35 g) pine nuts
¹/₂ tablespoon olive oil
1 tablespoon (15 ml) lemon juice
Salt and freshly ground black pepper, to taste

3 cups (201 g) baby kale, torn into bite-size pieces
¹/₂ cup (75 g) berries (I like raspberries, but blueberries, strawberries, and blackberries also work)

Place the pine nuts in a small skillet over medium-low heat and toast for about 3 minutes. When you do this, stand at the stove the whole time, stirring (or you *will* burn them!). Once they're lightly brown, remove them from the heat and transfer to a bowl so that the residual heat in the pan doesn't burn the nuts.

In a large bowl, add the oil, lemon juice, salt, pepper, and kale leaves. Massage the ingredients into the kale leaves for several minutes. Don't be gentle—the goal is to soften the kale. Place the bowl in the fridge and let it sit for 10 minutes. Mix in pine nuts and berries before serving.

YIELD: 4 SERVINGS

PER SERVING: 88 Calories; 6 g Fat (51.3% calories from fat); 3 g Protein; 8 g Carbohydrate; 3 g Dietary Fiber; 0 mg Cholesterol; 22 mg Sodium

SMOOTHIES, ENERGY BARS, AND FOOD FOR SPORTS

THE PERFECT SMOOTHIE FORMULA

When I first discovered smoothies as the perfect, high-energy, plant-based breakfast, I found a recipe I liked and drank that smoothie every single day. As you can guess, I got tired of that smoothie, and I realized I needed a better way, so I came up with The Perfect Smoothie Formula—just one recipe to remember and a different smoothie every day of your life. In addition to being composed almost entirely of raw fruits and vegetables, smoothies are great for serving as a vehicle for other nutritious ingredients. An example follows this recipe, or you can choose an ingredient from each category listed below (or feel free to use an ingredient we haven't listed). You can find several more ingredient suggestions and example recipes on my website: www.nomeatathlete.com/formulas.

1 soft fruit
2 small handfuls frozen or fresh fruit
2 to 4 tablespoons (16 to 32 g) protein powder
2 tablespoons binder

1¹⁄₂ tablespoons (23 ml) oil (optional)
1¹⁄₂ cups (355 ml) liquid
1 tablespoon sweetener, to taste
Superfood add-ins
6 ice cubes (omit if soft fruit is frozen)

Select one or more ingredients of each type and add to the blender in specified proportions. Blend until smooth. You may find that you need to use more or less water to get the consistency you like.

YIELD: 2 SMOOTHIES (16 ounces [475 ml] each)

PER SERVING (EXCLUDING UNKNOWN ITEMS): 390 Calories; 25 g Fat (53.1% calories from fat); 17 g Protein; 32 g Carbohydrate; 8 g Dietary Fiber; 25 mg Cholesterol; 65 mg Sodium

RECIPE NOTE

If you have a high-speed blender that can purée, say, a whole apple or carrot without leaving any chunks behind, then the purée of almost any fruit or vegetable can act as your soft fruit in this recipe.

SUGGESTIONS TO CREATE YOUR OWN SMOOTHIE

For each component of the Perfect Smoothie Formula, choose one or a combination of suggested ingredients below (or try one I haven't thought of!).

RECOMMENDED SOFT FRUITS
(choose 1)

Banana
Avocado

RECOMMENDED FRESH OR FROZEN FRUITS (2 small handfuls)

Strawberries (you can leave the greens on
   if you have a powerful blender)
Blueberries
Blackberries
Raspberries
Peaches
Mango
Pineapple

RECOMMENDED PROTEIN POWDERS
(2 to 4 tablespoons [16 to 36 g], a blend of all three is recommended)

Hemp
Sprouted brown rice (it tastes chalkier than
   hemp, but packs more protein per dollar)
Pea

RECOMMENDED BINDERS (2 tablespoons)

Ground flaxseed (14 g)
Almond butter or any nut butter (32 g)
Soaked raw almonds (soak for several hours
   and rinse before using) (18 g pre-soaked)
Rolled oats, whole or ground (10 g)
Udo's Wholesome Fast Food (16 g)
Raw Walnuts (13 g)

RECOMMENDED OILS
(optional, 1½ tablespoons)

Flaxseed oil (23 ml)
Udo's Blend or other essential fatty acid
   blend (23 ml)
Hemp oil (23 ml)
Virgin coconut oil (21 g)
Coconut butter (also called coconut
   manna, includes coconut flesh so is
   more a whole food than oil) (21 g)

RECOMMENDED LIQUIDS (1½ cups [355 ml])

Water (my favorite)
Almond milk or other nut milk
Hemp milk
Brewed tea
Brewed coffee

RECOMMENDED SWEETENERS
(optional, 1 tablespoon, or to taste)

Agave nectar (it's high in fructose, so choose this
   only before workouts) (20 g)
Stevia (the amount needed will vary by brand)
Lucuma powder (12 g)
Medjool dates, pitted (2 to 3 dates)
Maple syrup (20 g)

SUPERFOOD ADD-INS (optional, amounts vary)

Cacao nibs (1 to 2 tablespoons [8 to 16 g])
Carob chips (1 to 2 tablespoons [11 to 22 g])
Ground organic cinnamon (1 to 2 teaspoons
   [2.3 to 4.6 g])
Chia seeds, whole or ground (1 to 2 tablespoons
   [14 to 28 g])
Greens powder (1 to 2 teaspoons [2.6 to 5.3 g])
Whole spinach leaves (1 to 2 handfuls)
Maca powder (1 to 2 teaspoons [2.6 to 5.3 g])
Jalapeno pepper, seeds and stem removed (one
   small pepper)
Ground cayenne pepper (small pinch)
Sea salt (pinch)
Lemon or lime juice (1 tablespoon [15 ml])
Miso paste (1 teaspoon)
Raw pumpkin seeds, also called pepitas, shells
   removed (1 to 2 tablespoons [9 to 18 g])

EXAMPLE: EVERYDAY STRAWBERRY SMOOTHIE

1 banana

2 small handfuls frozen strawberries

4 tablespoons (24 g) hemp/rice/pea
protein powder blend

2 tablespoons (14 g) ground flaxseed

1 tablespoon (14 g) coconut butter

1¹/₂ cups (355 ml) water

1 tablespoon (20 g) maple syrup

1 handful fresh baby spinach

2 tablespoons (14 g) chia seeds

6 ice cubes

Combine all the ingredients in a blender and blend until smooth.

YIELD: 2 SMOOTHIES (16 ounces [475 ml] each)

PER SERVING (EXCLUDING UNKNOWN ITEMS): 456 Calories; 15 g Fat (27.2% calories from fat); 22 g Protein; 67 g Carbohydrate; 11 g Dietary Fiber; 49 mg Cholesterol; 87 mg Sodium

THE SIMPLEST HOMEMADE SPORTS DRINK

This ridiculously simple sports drink provides adequate hydration, sugar, and electrolytes for a workout, and it's what I most commonly make for my own runs. With most fruit juices, a 1:1 ratio of water to juice will give you 25 to 30 grams of carbohydrates per 16 ounces (475 ml), like most commercial sports drinks, but you can adjust the ratio depending on the sweetness of the juice you choose. Most fruit juices contain a decent amount of potassium, and adding ⅛ teaspoon of salt will get you 250 to 300 milligrams of sodium. The types of sugar in your juice (e.g., fructose, glucose, sucrose) do affect how quickly your body turns it into energy, but here, the point is simplicity.

1 cup (235 ml) water

1 cup (235 ml) natural fruit juice,
any kind

⅛ teaspoon sea salt

Combine the water with the fruit juice and stir in sea salt to dissolve.

YIELD: 1 DRINK (16 ounces [475 ml]) OR 2 DRINKS (8 ounces [235 ml])

Nutritional information will vary based on ingredients used.

A FANCIER SPORTS DRINK

This delicious sports drink recipe combines whole dates with maple syrup and a little bit of salt (for electrolytes) and lemon juice (to pack in a little more sugar and balance the sweetness of the dates and syrup). If desired, substitute coconut water for the water to add more potassium and other electrolytes as well as a different flavor. Because coconut water has sugar in it, you'll want to omit the maple syrup. Finally, use whole, fresh dates if you can find them, rather than the dried, packaged kind that come with the pits already removed—fresh dates blend with the other ingredients much more easily and taste better.

2 cups (475 ml) water, more to taste
2 fresh medjool dates, pits removed
1 teaspoon maple syrup

1 tablespoon (15 ml) lemon juice
1 teaspoon sea salt

Process all the ingredients in a food processor or high-speed blender. Strain through a metal strainer into a pitcher or bottle and discard any solids that remain in the strainer.

Two cups (475 ml) of water will produce a relatively sweet sports drink, but once you've blended everything together, you can dilute the drink as desired with more water.

YIELD: 16 OUNCES

PER SERVING: 153 Calories; trace Fat (0.1% calories from fat); trace Protein; 42 g Carbohydrate; 4 g Dietary Fiber; 0 mg Cholesterol; 485 mg Sodium

CHIA FRESCA (ISKIATE)

Chia seeds have become a popular health food for their hydration properties and high amounts of protein, fiber, and fatty acids—and thanks in no small part to the stories that abound about Aztec warriors eating them to sustain their energy for battle. This simple drink, called iskiate, is very similar to one that's still enjoyed by the Tarahumara, the Mexican tribe of amazing ultrarunners featured in Chris McDougall's book Born to Run. *I drink it in the morning before most races and long runs, as well as before heading out for a night on the town.*

10 ounces (285 ml) cold water
1 tablespoon (14 g) dry chia seeds
A few teaspoons (10 to 15 ml) lemon
   or lime juice

Agave nectar or unrefined sugar, to taste
   (optional)

Stir the chia seeds into the water; let them sit for about five minutes. Stir again.

Add citrus juice and agave to taste and stir to dissolve.

_____

YIELD: 1 DRINK

_____

PER SERVING: 56 Calories; 3 g Fat (43.4% calories from fat); 2 g Protein; 7 g Carbohydrate; trace Dietary Fiber; 0 mg Cholesterol; 13 mg Sodium

HOMEMADE ENERGY GEL

Most commercial gels aren't very appetizing, but they do a good job of cramming a lot of sugar (plus electrolytes) into a small space, making them convenient for a long run. Dates are a whole food that do a similar job, and what I most often use for fuel on runs, but they do take up slightly more space than a gel packet. This homemade gel is made entirely from natural foods, and will provide you with carbohydrates and electrolytes in a compact form. To bring it on your run, pour it into a gel flask or small zippered bags, the corner of which you can bite off before squeezing the gel into your mouth. You can store this gel in the refrigerator, in an airtight container, for three or four days.

1 tablespoon (12 g) chia seeds, ground
4 tablespoons (60 ml) water
4 fresh medjool dates, pits removed

3 tablespoons (45 ml) lemon juice
1 teaspoon sea salt
1 teaspoon blackstrap molasses

In a small bowl, stir the ground chia seeds into the water and then set aside to let a thick gel form, about five minutes.

Meanwhile, combine the remaining ingredients in a food processor or high-speed blender, running the motor for a few seconds to chop up the dates as well as possible. When the chia gel has thickened, add it to other ingredients in the processor or blender and process until you obtain a smooth, gel-like consistency.

YIELD: ⅔ CUP (150 g) (about 5 standard 1.1 ounce [30 g] gel packets)

PER SERVING: 158 Calories; 9 g Fat (47.7% calories from fat); 5 g Protein; 17 g Carbohydrate; 5 g Dietary Fiber; 0 mg Cholesterol; 674 mg Sodium

RECIPE NOTE

If at all possible, use whole, fresh dates here (the kind that come with the pits in them). They'll blend much more easily than dried, packaged dates will, and they taste much richer, too.

THE INCREDIBLE ENERGY BAR FORMULA

After falling in love with the "formula" concept after I first tried it with smoothies (page 106), I asked my sister to help me come up with a similar template that could be used to create endless varieties of energy bars. The result has been a huge hit on my blog, with readers every week leaving comments about the new combinations they've come up with. As with the other formulas in this book, simply choose an ingredient from each category of the master recipe below (or feel free to use an ingredient we haven't listed). An example follows, and you can find several more ingredient suggestions and example recipes at www.nomeatathlete.com/formulas.

1 tablespoon (15 ml) grapeseed oil (optional)

1 can (15½ ounces, or 440 g) or 1½ cups cooked beans, drained and rinsed

½ cup binder

¼ cup sweetener

¼ cup soft, sweet fruit

1 teaspoon extract (optional)

1 teaspoon dry spice (optional)

¼ teaspoon sea salt

1½ cups (120 g) oats (you can toast them if you want, but I can't tell the difference)

1 cup combination of dry base ingredients

1 cup add-ins

Preheat oven to 350°F (180°C or gas mark 4). Rub a 9 x 13-inch (23 x 33 cm) pan with grapeseed oil or grease with baking spray and set aside.

In a food processor, combine beans, binder, sweetener, soft sweet fruit, extract, dry spice, and salt until smooth. Add the oats and dry base ingredients and pulse just to combine. Add the add-ins and pulse again just to combine. If the consistency seems spreadable, you're good. If it's too dry, add ¼ cup (60 ml) of water. If it's too runny, add an additional ¼ cup of the dry base ingredient.

Spread mixture into oiled pan. Bake for 15 to 18 minutes. Cut into 24 bars.

YIELD: 24 BARS

Nutritional information will vary based on ingredients used.

SUGGESTIONS TO CREATE YOUR OWN ENERGY BAR

You'll have the most success if you use unsalted, unsweetened versions of the ingredients and control the sweetness and saltiness through the sweetener and added salt.

RECOMMENDED BEANS (15½ ounce or 440 g can, or 1½ cups cooked)

White beans (269 g)
Black beans (258 g)
Pinto beans (257 g)
Chickpeas (246 g)
Adzuki beans (345 g)

RECOMMENDED BINDER
(½ cup or amount specified below)

Almond butter (130 g)
Peanut butter (130 g)
¼ cup of ground flaxseed (28 g)
    mixed with ¼ cup (60 ml) water
Puréed pumpkin (120 g)
Mashed avocado (115 g)

RECOMMENDED SOFT, SWEET FRUIT
(¼ cup)

Applesauce (60 g)
Mashed banana (113 g) (about half of one)
Chopped dates (45 g) (remove the pits!)
Crushed pineapple (60 g)

RECOMMENDED SWEETENER
(¼ cup [80 g])

Maple syrup
Brown rice syrup
Agave nectar

RECOMMENDED OPTIONAL EXTRACT
(1 teaspoon [5 ml], optional)

Vanilla
Almond
Lemon
Coconut
Coffee

RECOMMENDED DRY SPICES
(1 teaspoon, optional)

Cinnamon
Ginger
Nutmeg*
Cardamom*
Instant coffee

*For stronger spices like nutmeg and cardamom, use just ¼ to ½ teaspoon and combine with less intense spices like cinnamon.

DRY BASE INGREDIENTS
(1 cup total, combination)

Protein powder (pea, hemp, and rice
    blend) (128 g)
Brown rice flour (160 g)
Spelt flour (140 g)
Cocoa (½ cup [40 g] maximum)
Whole wheat flour (120 g)
Buckwheat flour (120 g)

ADD-INS (1 cup)

Shredded coconut (85 g)
Dried cranberries (120 g)
Raisins (145 g)
Dried, diced apricots (130 g)
Chopped nuts (varies based on nut)
Cacao nibs (128 g)
Dry cereal (varies based on brand)
Chocolate chips (175 g)

EXAMPLE: CRANBERRY PISTACHIO PROTEIN BARS

1 tablespoon (15 ml) grapeseed oil, optional

1 can (15$^{1}/_{2}$ ounces, or 439 g) chickpeas, drained and rinsed

$^{1}/_{4}$ cup (28 g) ground flaxseed mixed with $^{1}/_{4}$ cup (60 ml) water

$^{1}/_{4}$ cup (80 g) agave nectar

$^{1}/_{4}$ cup (60 g) applesauce

1 teaspoon vanilla extract

1 teaspoon cinnamon

$^{1}/_{4}$ teaspoon salt

1$^{1}/_{2}$ cups (120 g) oats

1 cup (128 g) vanilla protein powder

$^{1}/_{2}$ cup (62 g) pistachios

$^{1}/_{2}$ cup (60) dried cranberries

Preheat oven to 350°F (180°C, or gas mark 4). Rub a 9 x 13-inch (23 x 33 cm) pan with grapeseed oil or grease with baking spray and set aside.

Follow recipe instructions in the master Incredible Energy Bar Formula using the ingredients listed above.

YIELD: 24 BARS

PER SERVING: 179 Calories; 5 g Fat (23.0% calories from fat); 11 g Protein; 24 g Carbohydrate; 6 g Dietary Fiber; 16 mg Cholesterol; 46 mg Sodium

CHOCOLATE QUINOA PROTEIN BARS

These delicious bars provide a boost of quick energy from the glucose in the dates, which your body begins using almost immediately after you eat them. But don't think these bars are all carbohydrates—the quinoa, flaxseed, protein powder, and optional nuts make these bars a perfect during- or post-workout snack.

³/₄ cup (128 g) dry quinoa, or about 2 cups (370 g) cooked

¹/₂ cup (89 g) dates, pitted

3 tablespoons (60 g) agave nectar

2 tablespoons (28 ml) grapeseed oil or melted coconut oil

2 tablespoons (14 g) ground flaxseed

¹/₂ teaspoon almond extract

¹/₄ teaspoon salt

¹/₂ cup (64 g) unsweetened protein powder (I like hemp protein the best here)

¹/₂ cup (60 g) whole wheat flour

¹/₂ cup add-ins, like dried fruit, nuts, shredded coconut, or vegan chocolate chips (I like half chocolate chips [44 g] and half dried shredded coconut [22 g])

Preheat oven to 350°F (180°C, or gas mark 4). Spray an 8-inch (20 cm) square baking dish lightly with baking spray or rub with coconut oil.

Rinse the dry quinoa in cold water and then let sit in a bowl of water for 10 minutes. In the meantime, bring 1 cup (235 ml) of water to boil. Drain the quinoa and add to the boiling water. Cover, reduce heat to simmer, and cook for about 12 minutes until quinoa is translucent and the water is absorbed. Let cool.

In the bowl of a food processor, combine the cooked quinoa, dates, agave nectar, grapeseed oil, flaxseed, almond extract, and salt. Process until relatively smooth (the quinoa will stay slightly lumpy). Transfer to a large bowl and set aside.

In a small bowl, stir together the protein powder, flour, and add-ins. Fold this dry mixture into the wet mixture.

Spread batter evenly in baking pan, pressing down with a spatula (the dough will be very thick, like cookie dough). Bake for about 22 to 25 minutes until firm. Let cool and then slice into 12 bars. Store in an airtight container for up to a week or freeze for up to three months.

YIELD: 12 BARS

PER SERVING (EXCLUDING UNKNOWN ITEMS): 201 Calories; 8 g Fat (34.6% calories from fat); 7 g Protein; 27 g Carbohydrate; 6 g Dietary Fiber; 0 mg Cholesterol; 72 mg Sodium

MOMO GRANOLA BARS

This is a DIY energy bar with whole ingredients at its base. It has enough carbs for a pre-workout pick-me-up, enough protein for a post-workout recovery, and enough great flavors for a dessert or snack anytime. —Mo Ferris, Johnson & Wales–trained chef and vegetarian marathoner

2 cups (160 g) rolled oats
¹/₂ cup (50 g) rough chopped roasted
   and salted almonds
¹/₄ cup (55 g) rough chopped pecans
¹/₂ cup (84 g) flaxseed
¹/₄ cup (16 g) raw pumpkin seeds

3 tablespoons (23 g) hemp seeds
¹/₂ cup (80 g) chopped dried cherries
2 small pinches kosher salt
¹/₃ cup (89 g) peanut butter
¹/₂ cup (172 g) brown rice syrup

Preheat oven to 350°F (180°C, or gas mark 4). Spread oats, almonds, pecans, flaxseed, pumpkin seeds, and hemp seeds onto an ungreased baking sheet and toast in the oven for 10 minutes. Gently shake and stir the oat mixture after 5 minutes to avoid burning the top layer and allowing both sides of the nuts and oats to brown.

Remove the mixture from oven and add to a large bowl, along with the cherries and salt. Decrease oven temperature to 300°F (150°C, or gas mark 2).

In a small saucepan, melt the peanut butter over medium-low heat, stirring constantly. Once the peanut butter is melted and slightly thinner, remove from heat and pour over oat mixture. Mix thoroughly.

In a separate small saucepan, add the brown rice syrup. Over medium-high heat, bring to a boil. When the bubbles that form get big and meet in the middle, immediately remove from heat, pour over the oat mixture, and thoroughly mix.

While still warm, pour the mixture out into the corner of a baking sheet lined with a silpat or parchment paper. Using wax paper, firmly press and spread mixture into the shape of a rectangle ¹/₄ inch (6 mm) thick (no gaps!). Note: The mixture will most likely not fill the entire sheet. Bake for 15 minutes or just until the edges begin to brown. Cool completely. Flip the rectangle out onto a cutting board and cut into 3 x 5 inch (7.5 x 13 cm) bars.

Wrap bars individually in plastic wrap and store in a large plastic bag.

YIELD: ABOUT 12 BARS

PER SERVING: 257 Calories; 15 g Fat (51.3% calories from fat); 8 g Protein; 25 g Carbohydrate; 6 g Dietary Fiber; 0 mg Cholesterol; 61 mg Sodium

SUPERFOOD ENERGY BARS

When my wife and I go on road trips with our kids, we make a huge batch of these bars ahead of time. Our son loves them, and if a toddler is going to stuff his face with energy bars, they might as well have beans and loads of superfoods in them! These bars are also excellent for fueling workouts or, better, for jump-starting the recovery process immediately afterward.

³/₄ cup (105 g) cornmeal or (87 g) masa harina

¹/₄ cup (32 g) maca root powder

¹/₂ cup (64 g) hemp protein powder

¹/₄ cup (56 g) chia seeds

2 tablespoons (14 g) ground flaxseed

1 tablespoon (7 g) ground cinnamon

1 teaspoon salt

2 cups (460 g) cooked adzuki or other beans

1 cup (178 g) or about 15 fresh medjool dates, chopped, pits removed

1¹/₂ cups (355 ml) water (you may substitute brewed yerba mate, green tea, or coffee)

¹/₄ cup (80 g) agave nectar or maple syrup

¹/₂ cup (130 g) natural nut butter

¹/₂ cup (125 g) unsweetened applesauce

¹/₄ cup (60 ml) fresh lime juice

1¹/₂ cups (28.5 g) puffed millet

1¹/₂ cups (150 g) raw almonds, chopped

Preheat the oven to 350°F (180°C, or gas mark 4). Grease a 9 x 13-inch (23 x 33 cm) casserole dish with baking spray or 1 tablespoon (15 ml) melted coconut oil or grapeseed oil.

In a medium-sized bowl, mix together the cornmeal, maca root powder, protein powder, chia seeds, ground flaxseed, cinnamon, and salt. Set aside.

In a food processor, puree the beans, dates, and water. If you've got room in your food processor, add the agave nectar or maple syrup, nut butter, applesauce, and lime juice and pulse to combine; otherwise, transfer the contents of the food processor to a large bowl and stir in those ingredients by hand. Stir in the cornmeal mixture. Fold in the puffed millet and almonds.

Spread the batter into the prepared pan. Bake for 30 to 35 minutes or until firm. Allow to cool and then cut into 24 bars. Store in an airtight container in the refrigerator.

YIELD: 24 BARS

PER SERVING: 192 Calories; 7 g Fat (32.0% calories from fat); 6 g Protein; 28 g Carbohydrate; 5 g Dietary Fiber; 0 mg Cholesterol; 112 mg Sodium

BUCKWHEAT PINOLE AND CHIA PANCAKES

In Chris McDougall's Born to Run, *pinole is described as toasted, ground corn and a food that the Tarahumara people use to fuel their runs by mixing with water into a paste or a drink. Although true pinole is made from nixtamalized maize (meaning the corn is soaked and cooked in an alkaline solution) found where the Tarahumara reside in Mexico, my sister Christine and I came up a version just about anyone can make using masa harina, a cornmeal that has undergone the same nixtamalization process as pinole and is usually used for making corn tortillas. These pancakes pack serious energy and are best before or during long runs.*

$^1/_2$ cup (58 g) masa harina or (70 g) fine-ground cornmeal

$^1/_4$ cup (56 g) chia seeds

$^1/_2$ cup (60 g) buckwheat flour

$^1/_2$ teaspoon salt

1 teaspoon baking powder

$^1/_4$ cup (60 g) applesauce

1 cup (235 ml) soy, almond, or hemp milk

2 tablespoons (28 ml) coconut oil, melted

2 tablespoons (40 g) maple syrup

1 teaspoon vanilla extract

Heat a large skillet over medium-high heat. Add masa harina or cornmeal and stir frequently until the color changes to a light brown, about 5 minutes. Remove from heat and let cool.

Stir together the toasted corn, chia seeds, buckwheat flour, salt, and baking powder in a large bowl. Whisk in the applesauce, milk, melted coconut oil, maple syrup, and vanilla extract.

Heat a medium-sized skillet over medium heat. Grease lightly with baking spray. Pour about $^1/_4$ cup (28 g) of batter into pan and tilt the pan to spread the batter evenly. Cook for 3 to 4 minutes, flipping halfway through (it should be easy to slide the spatula under the pancake when it's time to flip).

Repeat with remaining batter, greasing the pan between each pancake as needed.

YIELD: 6 LARGE PANCAKES

PER SERVING: 191 Calories; 8 g Fat (35.5% calories from fat); 5 g Protein; 27 g Carbohydrate; 3 g Dietary Fiber; 0 mg Cholesterol; 180 mg Sodium

MAIN-EVENT MEALS

QUINOA WITH CASHEWS AND ORANGES

Quinoa is often mistakenly called a grain, but it's technically a seed, making it an excellent, higher-protein substitute for rice that's gluten-free as well. Quinoa is coated with a bitter substance called saponin that you'll need to rinse off before you use it. Quinoa can be cooked ahead of time, frozen, and thawed prior to use. We often parcel out serving-size portions of cooked beans and grains on weekends and freeze them for use during the week.

1 cup (173 g) uncooked quinoa

2 tablespoons (28 ml) grapeseed oil, divided

1 small onion, finely chopped

1 can (11 ounces, or 310 g) mandarin oranges, juice reserved, or 2 fresh oranges, peeled, segments chopped in half

Enough water to bring total amount of liquid from oranges to 2 cups (475 ml) (the amount will vary depending on choice of canned or fresh oranges)

1/2 cup (70 g) raw cashews, chopped

1 bag (16 ounces, or 455 g) frozen stir-fry vegetables

1/4 cup (60 ml) rice wine (you can substitute another cooking wine)

1/4 cup (60 ml) tamari

1 clove garlic, minced

1 tablespoon (8 g) cornstarch or arrowroot

Rinse the quinoa in cold water. Let sit in cold water and set aside.

Heat 1 tablespoon (15 ml) of the oil over medium heat in a medium saucepan. Add the onion and stir occasionally until translucent but not brown, 5 to 7 minutes.

Drain the quinoa and rinse one more time. Then add to the saucepan and stir for a minute to lightly toast. Add the 2 cups (475 ml) of liquid (water or water plus orange juice), bring to a boil, and reduce heat to medium-low. Cover the pan and simmer for about 15 minutes until the water is absorbed and the quinoa is tender. Remove from the heat and fluff with a fork.

While the quinoa cooks, lightly toast the cashews in a dry skillet over medium-low heat. Stir frequently for 3 to 5 minutes until cashews are golden but not brown. Transfer to a plate and set aside.

Heat the remaining tablespoon (15 ml) of oil over medium-high heat in a large skillet. Add the frozen vegetables and stir occasionally until tender-crisp, 5 to 8 minutes.

(continued on next page)

While the vegetables cook, whisk together the rice wine, tamari, garlic, and cornstarch in a bowl. When the vegetables are ready, pour the rice wine mixture into the pan and stir for a minute or so to cook off the alcohol.

Fold the cooked quinoa, cashews, and oranges into the vegetables and serve.

YIELD: 4 SERVINGS

PER SERVING (EXCLUDING UNKNOWN ITEMS): 435 Calories; 18 g Fat (36.8% calories from fat); 14 g Protein; 55 g Carbohydrate; 8 g Dietary Fiber; 0mg Cholesterol; 1039 mg Sodium

TOMATO AND WHITE BEAN RISOTTO

The Cashew "Cheese" Spread and Sauce (page 145) in this dish is optional but highly recommended; it makes a creamy risotto even creamier. If you aren't using the cashew cheese, add a few tablespoons (28 to 45 ml) of olive oil just before the risotto is done instead or just skip this step entirely.

6 cups (1.4 L) vegetable stock (a combination of vegetable stock and water is okay, too)
¼ cup (60 ml) extra virgin olive oil
1 small onion, diced small
1 tablespoon (1.7 g) chopped fresh rosemary, divided into 3 teaspoons
1 tablespoon (2.4 g) chopped fresh thyme
Small pinch crushed red pepper flakes
2 cups (460 g) uncooked Arborio rice
½ cup (120 ml) dry wine, white or red

2 cups (490 g) Tasty Three-Ingredient Tomato Sauce (page 144) or prepared tomato sauce
1 can (15 ounces, or 425 g) white beans, drained and rinsed
½ cup (115 g) Cashew "Cheese" Spread and Sauce (page 145), made to a spread consistency (optional)
Sea salt and fresh ground black pepper, to taste

In a medium-size pot, bring the vegetable stock to a slow simmer.

Heat the olive oil in a large pot over high heat. Add the onion and cook for 2 minutes, stirring frequently. Add 1 teaspoon of the rosemary, the thyme, and the red pepper flakes and cook for another minute.

Add the rice to the pan and toast, stirring frequently for 2 to 3 minutes. Pour in the wine and stir until it evaporates. Then add 3 cups (700 ml) of the simmering vegetable stock along with the tomato sauce.

Stir vigorously for 30 seconds and then stop. Allow the liquid to come to a boil and then reduce the heat to medium to maintain a steady bubbling. Stir only often enough to keep the rice from sticking to the bottom of the pan until all of the liquid has evaporated or been absorbed by the rice, about 10 to 12 minutes.

Add the rest of the simmering vegetable stock, stir for another 30 seconds, and then allow it to evaporate and absorb again, stirring only when necessary to prevent sticking.

The risotto is finished when there is just a tiny bit of firmness in the center of each grain of rice, and the risotto has a texture somewhere between that of mashed potatoes and thick soup. (If you find the liquid has evaporated before the rice is done, add water or stock, 1/2 cup [120 ml] at a time, stirring for a few seconds after each addition.) Just before it seems done, add the beans, stir, and allow them to heat through.

Remove from the heat and stir in another teaspoon of the rosemary and 2 tablespoons (29 g) of the cashew cheese. Add salt and pepper to taste.

Serve immediately, garnishing each bowl with the remaining rosemary and a dollop of cashew cheese in the center.

YIELD: 5 TO 6 SERVINGS

PER SERVING: 875 Calories; 26 g Fat (27.4% calories from fat); 30 g Protein; 128 g Carbohydrate; 16 g Dietary Fiber; 2 mg Cholesterol; 2098 mg Sodium

RECIPE VARIATION

Arborio rice is the traditional risotto rice, but it's more processed than what I usually like to eat. (I save this recipe for carbo-loading meals.) If you prefer, you can replace the rice with barley for a healthier everyday version, though this will add a significant amount of cooking time and the risotto won't have quite the decadent texture it usually does.

WHITE BEAN COCONUT CURRY

Anjum's New Indian, by Anjum Anand, is the book that introduced me to the fabulous world of Indian cooking (the book is not vegetarian, but it has a nice section on vegetables and lentil and bean dishes). Before reading this book, I had assumed those deep, spicy flavors were strictly the domain of restaurants with tandoor ovens, but it turns out you can come remarkably close with just a few spices and the equipment in your own kitchen. This mildly sweet, coconutty bean curry is inspired by a recipe in that book, made vegan and slightly simplified.

2 tablespoons (28 g) coconut or
    grapeseed oil (28 ml)
1 teaspoon mustard seeds, brown or yellow
10 fresh basil leaves
1 small onion, diced
$\frac{1}{2}$-inch (1.3 cm) piece of fresh ginger,
    peeled and minced
3 cloves garlic, minced
1 tablespoon (6.3 g) curry powder
$\frac{1}{2}$ teaspoon salt, more to taste

1 can (13$\frac{1}{2}$ ounces, or 400 ml) light
    coconut milk, shaken
1 can (15 ounces, or 425 g) or 1$\frac{1}{2}$ cups
    (269 g) white beans, any variety,
    drained and rinsed
1 pint grape tomatoes
1$\frac{1}{2}$ teaspoons brown sugar
Juice of $\frac{1}{2}$ lemon
Shredded coconut and chopped fresh
    basil or cilantro, for garnish

Heat the oil in a large saucepan over medium heat. Add the mustard seeds and basil leaves and after a minute, add the onion. Cook, stirring occasionally, for 6 to 8 minutes, allowing the onion to lightly brown. Add the ginger and garlic and cook for 30 seconds or so until fragrant. Then add the curry powder and salt and cook for another 30 seconds. (You don't want the garlic to brown; have the coconut milk open and ready to pour so that it won't.)

Add the coconut milk, stir, and raise the heat to high. After it boils, reduce heat to medium and add the beans, tomatoes, and brown sugar. Allow everything to simmer for 5 minutes or so and then stir in the lemon juice and season with more salt and more lemon juice to taste.

Garnish with coconut and basil or cilantro and serve.

YIELD: 4 SERVINGS

PER SERVING: 520 Calories; 14 g Fat (22.4% calories from fat); 28 g Protein; 78 g Carbohydrate; 18 g Dietary Fiber; 0 mg Cholesterol; 318 mg Sodium

PASTA WITH ROASTED TOMATOES, CHICKPEAS, AND ARUGULA

The oven-roasted tomatoes absolutely make this dish! They take 45 minutes to roast, but you can perform the rest of steps in the recipe while they're cooking, so total preparation time isn't much more than that.

3 pounds (1.4 Kg) medium plum tomatoes, halved lengthwise
2 cloves garlic, minced
1 tablespoon (6 g) Italian seasoning
1/4 to 1/2 teaspoon crushed red pepper
1/4 cup (60 ml) plus 1 tablespoon (15 ml) olive or grapeseed oil, divided
Sea salt and black pepper, to taste
6 quarts (5.7 L) water
2 tablespoons (30 g) sea salt
12 ounces (340 g) whole wheat or alternative grain pasta, any shape
1 can (14 1/2 ounces, 410 g) or 1 1/2 cups (246 g) cooked chickpeas, drained and rinsed
4 cups (80 g) lightly packed arugula
Zest of 1 lemon (plus juice, optional, for serving)

Preheat the oven to 400°F (200°C, or gas mark 6).

Spread out the tomatoes on a foil-lined baking pan. Mix together the garlic, Italian seasoning, red pepper, 1/4 cup (60 ml) of oil, and a few pinches of salt and pepper and then pour the mixture evenly over tomatoes. Roast in the oven until soft and lightly browned, about 45 minutes. When the tomatoes have finished roasting, crush half of the roasted tomatoes in a large bowl with a fork and set aside.

Add water and 2 tablespoons (30 g) of salt to a large pot and bring to a boil. Add pasta and cook until al dente, according to package instructions. Reserve 1/4 cup (60 ml) of the pasta water to thin the sauce if needed.

While the pasta cooks, heat the remaining oil over medium heat in a medium-sized pan. Add the chickpeas and arugula to the pan. Once the chickpeas are heated through and the arugula is wilted, add them to the crushed tomatoes in the bowl, along with the cooked pasta and lemon zest, and then toss to mix. Add the reserved pasta water as needed to thin the sauce.

Divide the pasta among four plates, top with the remaining roasted tomatoes, and add salt, pepper, and lemon juice to taste.

YIELD: 4 SERVINGS

PER SERVING: 670 Calories; 20 g Fat (25.2% calories from fat); 25 g Protein; 108 g Carbohydrate; 14 g Dietary Fiber; 0 mg Cholesterol; 91 mg Sodium

PASTA WITH PESTO, POTATOES, AND GREEN BEANS

For several years, this traditional Italian dish has been my go-to carbo-loading meal the day before races. The potatoes and pasta provide the carbs, the beans add protein, and the pesto just makes it all delicious. Pesto is typically made with pine nuts, which are expensive, and often with cheese. Here, we use raw almonds instead of pine nuts, but just about any nut will work. Lemon juice isn't a typical pesto ingredient, but helps give the pesto a bright, acidic bite and works nicely with the other summer flavors. Note: To save time, make the pesto while the vegetables and pasta cook.

FOR THE VEGETABLES AND PASTA:

4 or 5 medium-small boiling potatoes, peeled and cut into 1-inch (2.5 cm) chunks

2 tablespoons (30 g) sea salt

1¼ cups (125 g) fresh green beans, trimmed and cut into 1 inch (2.5 cm) lengths

16 ounces (455 g) whole wheat pasta, any shape (I like trenette or penne)

Juice of half a lemon

Salt and fresh ground black pepper, to taste

FOR THE PESTO:

2 cups (80 g) or one large bunch fresh basil, thickest stems removed

⅓ cup (48 g) raw almonds (walnuts or pine nuts work, too)

1 clove garlic, peeled

2 tablespoons (28 ml) lemon juice

Sea salt, to taste

⅓ cup (80 ml) good-quality olive oil

1 tablespoon (15 ml) almond or soy milk, or reserved pasta-cooking water (to thin the pesto, as needed)

To make the vegetables and pasta: Place the potatoes in a large pot (you'll be using it for the pasta, too) and fill with as much water as you'd use to make the pasta. (You want to at least cover the potatoes by an inch or two, but you'll probably need more than this for the pasta.)

Add the salt to the water and bring to a boil. When the potatoes are a few minutes from being tender, around 8 to 10 minutes, add the green beans to the boiling water.

Cook for another 3 to 5 minutes until the green beans and potatoes are tender and then remove them with a slotted spoon and transfer to a separate bowl. Cover with foil or the lid of a pot to keep warm.

Put the pasta into the boiling water and cook until al dente. Reserve ¹/₂ cup (120 ml) of the pasta water, in case you need it to loosen the pesto.

To make the pesto: Combine basil, nuts, garlic, lemon juice, and a pinch of salt in a food processor and pulse until it becomes a coarse paste. With the machine running, drizzle in the olive oil and let it process until the mixture is relatively smooth. Add salt to taste. Before adding to pasta or other dishes, stir in the almond or soy milk or reserved pasta water to thin it a bit.

Place the pasta, potatoes, and green beans in a large bowl. Mix in the pesto to coat everything, gradually adding more liquid to achieve desired consistency. Add lemon juice, salt, and pepper to taste.

YIELD: 6 SERVINGS

PER SERVING: 430 Calories; 10 g Fat (19.4% calories from fat); 15 g Protein; 77 g Carbohydrate; 10 g Dietary Fiber; 0 mg Cholesterol; 1895 mg Sodium

RECIPE SUGGESTIONS

Although pesto is called for in only one recipe in this book, its uses are endless. You can toss it with pasta or gnocchi, spread it on pizza dough or flatbread, mix it with Cashew "Cheese" Spread and Sauce (page 145), dip vegetables in it, stir it into olive oil for a great bread dipper, smear it across a plate to give a dish a little flair, or put a dollop in the middle of your risotto.

SUPER QUICK RED LENTILS AND RICE

Although this dish takes about half an hour to simmer, the active cooking time is less than two minutes! Most of these ingredients should be staples in your pantry, and if you don't happen to have the spinach or cilantro on hand, they can both be omitted. The spices are my attempt to replicate the Indian combination known as panch phoran *using common spices found in most grocery stores.*

2¹/₂ cups (480 g) red lentils, rinsed under cold water until it runs clear
6 cups (1.4 L) water
1 teaspoon ground turmeric
1¹/₂ teaspoons chili powder
1¹/₂ teaspoons salt
2 tablespoons (28 g) coconut or grapeseed oil (28 ml)
1 teaspoon fennel seed
1¹/₂ teaspoons cumin seed
1¹/₂ teaspoons dried marjoram or oregano

1¹/₂ teaspoons mustard seed
¹/₄ teaspoon crushed red pepper flakes, more to taste
4 cups (120 g) baby spinach
¹/₂ cup (8 g) fresh cilantro, chopped
Lemon juice, for serving
Hot sauce, for serving (optional)
6 to 8 cups (62 to 1.6 Kg) cooked brown rice, or Simple Indian Street Bread (page 146), for serving

Combine the lentils and water in a large pot and stir in the turmeric, chili powder, and salt. Bring to a boil over high heat and then reduce heat to medium and simmer, uncovered, stirring occasionally until the lentils are tender and the mixture is more or less homogeneous, 25 to 30 minutes. (Some of the lentils will dissolve completely while others will just barely hold their shape and provide some texture.)

When the lentils are about 2 minutes from being done, heat the oil in a separate pan over medium-high heat. Add the fennel and cumin seed, marjoram, mustard seed, and red pepper flakes and stir for a minute. Then pour the spice-and-oil mixture into the pot with the lentils, along with the baby spinach, and stir to combine and wilt the spinach.

Serve over brown rice or alongside Simple Indian Street Bread (page 146), garnished with cilantro, lemon juice, hot sauce, and more salt to taste.

When reheating this dish (or if it sits for a while on the stove and begins to dry out), simply add some hot water and it will be like new again!

YIELD: ABOUT 6 SERVINGS

PER SERVING: 371 Calories; 7 g Fat (17.1% calories from fat); 13 g Protein; 65 g Carbohydrate; 11 g Dietary Fiber; 0 mg Cholesterol; 568 mg Sodium

PLANT RESTAURANT'S CURRIED LENTILS

Lentils are some of the most restorative, nutrient-dense foods an athlete can eat. The protein, iron, and fiber content of lentils make them a perfect staple. In this recipe, onions and ginger are puréed before being fried with garlic. This lends a smooth, rich texture to the final dish, which elevates the aromatic sauce and allows for the release of flavor. —Jason Sellers, chef and co-owner of Plant Restaurant, Asheville, North Carolina

2 tablespoons (12 g) ginger, roughly chopped

⅓ large yellow onion, roughly chopped

2 cups (384 g) of your favorite lentils

1 bay leaf

1 teaspoon salt

2 tablespoons (28 ml) safflower oil

¼ cup (40 g) minced garlic

3 tablespoons (19 g) curry powder or (21 g) garam masala

¼ cup (65 g) tomato paste

2 tablespoons (28 ml) lemon juice

2 cups (475 ml) coconut milk

1 cup (235 ml) vegetable stock or sodium-free broth

Salt, to taste

Add the ginger and onion to a blender and purée into a paste. Set aside.

Add the lentils and bay leaf to a stockpot, cover with water or vegetable stock, cover the pot and bring to a boil. Lower the heat and simmer until tender, about 25 to 30 minutes. Before the lentils are completely cooked, add the teaspoon of salt. Drain the lentils.

While lentils are cooking, combine safflower oil and garlic in a heavy-bottomed stock pot and cook garlic for 5 minutes over medium heat. (Don't let the garlic burn—if it's starting to, proceed immediately to the next step.) Add the onion-ginger paste and cook for 10 minutes until visibly drier. Stir in the curry powder or garam masala and tomato paste and cook for a couple of minutes until the mixture releases some of the oil. Lower the heat, add the lemon juice, coconut milk, vegetable stock, and salt, and stir to combine. Pour the mixture over the lentils and mix to make uniform.

YIELD: 8 SERVINGS

PER SERVING: 380 Calories; 19 g Fat (43.1% calories from fat); 17 g Protein; 40 g Carbohydrate; 18 g Dietary Fiber; trace Cholesterol; 551 mg Sodium

BIBIMBAP
(Korean Vegetables with Rice)

Bibimbap is a traditional one-dish Korean lunch of warm rice topped with raw or cooked vegetables, such as cucumbers, spinach, and soybean sprouts. Any vegetables, especially ones in season or perhaps left over from another recipe, will be great in this dish. —Mo Ferris, Johnson & Wales–trained chef and vegetarian marathoner

FOR THE SAUCE:

4 tablespoons (60 g) Korean chili paste, called gochujang, or another chili paste
2 tablespoons (28 ml) toasted sesame oil
1 tablespoon (15 ml) soy sauce or tamari
½ tablespoon sriracha
1 clove garlic, minced

FOR THE BIBIMBAP:

8 small carrots with tops, cut in half lengthwise and then in 3 inch (7.5 cm) pieces
2¼ cups (160 g) broccoli florets

4 stalks bok choy, cut in 2 inch (5 cm) pieces, leaves discarded
1 tablespoon (15 ml) olive oil
10 shiitake mushrooms, stems removed, cut in thirds
Salt and fresh ground black pepper, to taste
1 teaspoon toasted sesame oil
½ cup (75 g) fresh fava beans, cleaned
¾ cup fresh (150 g) or frozen (130 g) peas (ideally English peas)
2 cups (390 g) cooked brown rice
2 scallions, cut on a thin bias, for garnish
2 tablespoons (16 g) white sesame seeds, for garnish

Combine all the sauce ingredients in a small food processor and set aside.

Place the carrots, broccoli, and bok choy into a steamer basket in a medium pot with 1 to 2 inches (2.5 to 5 cm) of water and steam until slightly tender but still crunchy, about 4 minutes.

Heat a large sauté pan over medium-high heat, add olive oil and mushrooms, and sauté until very tender, 3 to 5 minutes. Season with salt and pepper. Remove mushrooms from pan. Add sesame oil to the pan and sauté carrots, broccoli, bok choy, fava beans, and peas over medium-high heat. Cook vegetables until they have a little color but are still crunchy, about 5 minutes. Place a cup (195 g) of the cooked brown rice into each of two serving bowls and mix with 1 to 2 tablespoons of sauce each. Add a mixture of the vegetables to the bowl and garnish with scallions and white sesame seeds.

YIELD: 2 SERVINGS

PER SERVING: 897 Calories; 32 g Fat (30.6% calories from fat); 30 g Protein; 133 g Carbohydrate; 32 g Dietary Fiber; 0 mg Cholesterol; 952 mg Sodium

CITRUS "COOKED" VEGGIES WITH ORZO

This delicious carbo-loader dish was inspired by a recipe from a Williams-Sonoma book simply called Pasta, *and that's exactly what orzo is, despite the grains being the same shape and size as rice. If you can get whole wheat orzo, feel free to use it. You can also use barley for a healthier version, though cooking time will be much longer and the texture of the final dish not quite as appealing.*

¹/₂ cup (60 ml) olive oil, divided
2 pints (600 g) cherry tomatoes, halved
   or quartered
1 clove garlic, minced
1 large or 2 small shallots, thinly sliced
1 jalapeño pepper, seeded and minced
Juice of 1 orange
Zest of 1 lemon

Salt, to taste
16 ounces (455 g) orzo
2 avocados, pitted, peeled, and diced
¹/₂ cup (130 g) Cashew "Cheese" Spread
   and Sauce (page 145, optional)
2 tablespoons (8 g) fresh oregano,
   chopped

In a large bowl, combine half of the oil, the tomatoes, garlic, shallots, jalapeño, orange juice, lemon zest, and a few generous pinches of salt. The salt will draw out the juice of the tomatoes to form a dressing. Let it sit while you prepare the orzo and the avocado.

Bring a large pot of water to a boil and then salt the water and add orzo. Cook for 8 to 10 minutes until al dente (don't overcook).

When the orzo is done, drain with a fine strainer and add it, along with the avocados, cashew cheese, and remaining oil to the bowl with the dressing and tomatoes. Mix everything well, being careful not to smash all the avocado pieces. Add the oregano and salt to taste.

YIELD: 6 SERVINGS

PER SERVING: 547 Calories; 25 g Fat (39.6% calories from fat); 14 g Protein; 71 g Carbohydrate; 5 g Dietary Fiber; 0 mg Cholesterol; 115 mg Sodium

BASIC BEANS AND RICE

Although this recipe is not quite a formula per se, *like the three true formula recipes in this book, hearty beans and rice are such a staple in my diet and that of many other vegan athletes that they warrant an abundance of recipe options (gotta keep it fresh!). Use this recipe to prepare the beans for each of the subsequent variations and to choose seasonings, garnishes, and the type of bean according to the variation you're making.*

1 tablespoon (15 ml) grapeseed oil
1 onion, chopped
1 clove garlic, minced
1 can (15½ ounces, or 440 g) or 1½ cups
 (257 g) cooked beans, drained and rinsed

Salt and freshly ground black pepper,
 to taste
2 cups (390 g) cooked brown rice

Heat the oil in a large pan over medium-high heat. Add the onion and cook until softened, about 5 minutes. Add the garlic and sauté for an additional 5 minutes, stirring often to avoid burning.

Stir in the beans. If cooking one of the variations, at this point you'll add ingredients and follow the instructions specific to that particular variation. Otherwise, heat beans through and season with salt and pepper to taste. Serve with rice.

YIELD: 4 SERVINGS

PER SERVING (excluding unknown items): 240 Calories; 5 g Fat (17.1% calories from fat); 8 g Protein; 42 g Carbohydrate; 6 g Dietary Fiber; 0 mg Cholesterol; 383 mg Sodium

RECIPE NOTE

It's worth noting, because it's so often mentioned, that the amino acids in beans and rice do, in fact, combine to form what's called a complete protein, meaning that all 9 essential amino acids are present in significant quantities. Although it's great to know you're getting all of the amino acids in a single meal, this actually isn't quite as important as it sounds because our bodies pool the amino acids we get throughout the day (see chapter 3 for more information). Nonetheless, beans and rice are a classic combination and a tasty way to get all of that protein.

EXAMPLE 1: INDIAN BEANS AND RICE WITH GINGER AND FRESH CILANTRO

1 recipe Basic Beans and Rice, prepared using chickpeas (page 130)

1 tablespoon (6.3 g) curry powder

1/2 teaspoon ground cinnamon

Thumb-sized piece fresh ginger, peeled and minced

1 can (15 ounces, or 425 g) diced tomatoes with green chilies, undrained

Salt and pepper, to taste

1/4 cup (4 g) chopped fresh cilantro

Prepare the Basic Beans and Rice recipe with chickpeas in a large pan. Stir the curry powder and cinnamon into the chickpea mixture. Sauté for a minute and then add the ginger and tomatoes and their juices. Cook on medium-high heat for 5 minutes until the tomatoes no longer taste raw.

Remove from the heat and add salt and pepper to taste. Stir the cilantro into the rice before serving with the beans.

YIELD: 4 SERVINGS

PER SERVING: 349 Calories; 5 g Fat (13.3% calories from fat); 15 g Protein; 63 g Carbohydrate; 11 g Dietary Fiber; 0 mg Cholesterol; 371 mg Sodium

FEELING-FANCY VERSION

Serve with Simple Indian Street Bread (page 146) and a side of sliced mangoes.

EXAMPLE 2: MEXICAN GREEN CHILE BEANS AND RICE

1 recipe Basic Beans and Rice, prepared
  using pinto beans (page 130)
2 teaspoons cumin
1 teaspoon chili powder
1 can (15 ounces, or 425 g) diced tomatoes
  with green chili peppers, drained

Juice of $\frac{1}{2}$ lime
Salt and pepper, to taste
$\frac{1}{4}$ cup (4 g) fresh chopped cilantro

Prepare the Basic Beans and Rice recipe using pinto beans in a large pan. Stir the cumin and chili powder into the beans and sauté for a minute to coat. Add the can of tomatoes and cook on medium-high heat for 5 minutes until the tomatoes no longer taste raw.

Remove from the heat, stir in the lime juice, and add salt and pepper to taste. Stir the cilantro into the rice before serving with the beans.

YIELD: 4 SERVINGS

PER SERVING (excluding unknown items): 273 Calories; 5 g Fat (16.8% calories from fat); 10 g Protein; 49 g Carbohydrate; 8 g Dietary Fiber; 0 mg Cholesterol; 402 mg Sodium

FEELING-FANCY VERSION
Serve with a side of sliced avocado and warm corn tortillas.

EXAMPLE 3: ASIAN ADZUKI BEANS AND RICE

1 recipe Basic Beans and Rice, prepared using adzuki or black beans (page 130)

4 medium carrots, peeled and cut into thin strips

Thumb-size piece fresh ginger, peeled and minced

2 tablespoons (28 ml) reduced-sodium soy sauce or tamari

1 can (11 ounces, or 310 g) mandarin oranges, juice reserved

Salt and pepper, to taste

1/2 teaspoon Chinese five spice powder

Prepare the Basic Beans and Rice using adzuki or black beans in a large pan. Sauté the carrots and ginger with the beans for a few minutes until the carrots are cooked but still crunchy. Stir in the soy sauce and 2 tablespoons (28 ml) of the reserved mandarin orange juice.

Remove from the heat and gently stir in the mandarin orange slices. Add salt and pepper to taste. Stir the Chinese five spice powder into the rice before serving with the beans.

YIELD: 4 SERVINGS

PER SERVING: 384 Calories; 5 g Fat (12.1% calories from fat); 15 g Protein; 72 g Carbohydrate; 12 g Dietary Fiber; 0 mg Cholesterol; 535 mg Sodium

FEELING-FANCY VERSION

Throw in some chopped cabbage, thinly sliced green bell pepper, and mushrooms with the carrots. Drizzle with hoisin sauce to serve.

EXAMPLE 4: HAWAIIAN LUAU BEANS AND RICE

1 recipe Basic Beans and Rice, prepared using black beans (page 130)

2 cups (180 g) chopped red cabbage (about quarter of a head)

1 can (20 ounces, or 560 g) sliced pineapple rings, juice reserved

2 tablespoons (28 ml) soy sauce or tamari, divided

3/4 teaspoon smoked paprika

2 cups (60 g) fresh baby spinach

Salt and pepper, to taste

1 teaspoon coconut oil

Prepare the Basic Beans and Rice using black beans in a large pan. Stir the red cabbage, 1/2 cup (120 ml) of the reserved pineapple juice, 1 tablespoon (15 ml) of the soy sauce, and smoked paprika into the beans. Cook for 5 minutes until the cabbage is cooked but still crunchy.

Stir in the spinach and cook for 2 more minutes until slightly wilted. Add salt and pepper to taste.

Meanwhile, melt the coconut oil in a large skillet over medium-high heat. Lay three-quarters of the pineapple rings in the pan and sprinkle with remaining 1 tablespoon (15 ml) of soy sauce or tamari (save the leftover rings for dessert!). Cook for 2 minutes per side until nice and charred. Serve on top of the beans along with the rice.

YIELD: 4 SERVINGS

PER SERVING: 423 Calories; 6 g Fat (13.1% calories from fat); 15 g Protein; 80 g Carbohydrate; 11 g Dietary Fiber; 0 mg Cholesterol; 527 mg Sodium

FEELING-FANCY VERSION

Add a chopped red bell pepper in with the cabbage, sprinkle beans with a minced jalapeño pepper, and fold 1/2 cup (43 g) toasted coconut into the cooked rice.

THE INCREDIBLE VEGGIE BURGER FORMULA

After the success of The Perfect Smoothie Formula (page 106) and The Incredible Energy Bar Formula (page 112), my sister Christine and I decided to complete the trifecta with what might just be the most useful formula of the bunch. Why a veggie burger formula? Because on those nights when it seems like you don't have the ingredients to make anything, I'd be willing to bet that with the help of this formula, you've got what it takes to throw together a mean veggie burger—without setting foot outside your house. An example follows, or you can choose an ingredient from each category listed on the next page (or feel free to use one we haven't listed). You can find several more ingredient suggestions and example recipes at www.nomeatathlete.com/formulas.

2 tablespoons (28 ml) plus 2 teaspoons oil, divided
½ cup (80 g) chopped onion
1 clove garlic, minced
2 cups diced veggies
1 can (15½ ounces, 440 g) or 1½ cups cooked beans, drained and rinsed

3 tablespoons (45 ml) liquid flavor
4 teaspoons spice
½ teaspoon (3 g) kosher salt (omit or reduce if liquid or spices contain salt)
1 cup dry base ingredient
½ cup texture ingredient

Heat 2 teaspoons oil in a large pan over medium heat. Sauté the onion, garlic, and veggies until softened, about 5 minutes.

Transfer to a food processor and pulse with the beans, liquid flavor, spice(s), and salt until combined but still chunky. Pulse in the dry base and texture ingredients. Form into golf ball size balls and flatten into patties.

Heat 2 tablespoons (28 ml) oil over medium-high heat in a large pan. Sauté the patties in batches for 2 to 3 minutes per side until browned and heated through.

YIELD: ABOUT 18 SMALL PATTIES (5-6 DINNER-SIZED SERVINGS)

Nutritional information will vary based on ingredients used.

SUGGESTIONS TO CREATE YOUR OWN VEGGIE BURGER

For each component of the Incredible Veggie Burger Formula on the previous page, choose one or a combination of suggested ingredients below (or try one we haven't thought of!).

RECOMMENDED OILS OR ALTERNATIVES (2 tablespoons [28 ml] plus 2 teaspoons)

Olive
Grapeseed
Coconut
Vegetable broth or water

RECOMMENDED DICED VEGGIES (2 cups)

Carrots (260 g)
Celery (200 g)
Mushrooms (140 g)
Chopped spinach (60 g)
Chopped kale (134 g)
Corn (300 g)
Chopped canned artichokes (600 g)
Zucchini (240 g)
Yellow squash (240 g)

RECOMMENDED BEANS (15½ ounces, or 440 g can or 1½ cups cooked)

White beans (269 g)
Black beans (258 g)
Pinto beans (257 g)
Chickpeas (246 g)
Adzuki beans (345 g)
Lentils (396 g)

RECOMMENDED LIQUID FLAVOR INGREDIENTS (3 tablespoons total; a combination is usually best)

Mustard (33 g)
Ketchup (45 g)
Soy sauce (45 ml)
Teriyaki sauce (45 ml)
Vegan Worcestershire sauce (45 ml)
Vegan buffalo sauce (48 g)
Balsamic vinegar (45 ml)
Salsa (49 g)
Pasta sauce (46 g)
Water (45 ml)
Liquid smoke (45 ml)

RECOMMENDED SPICES (4 teaspoons total; a combination is usually best)

Smoked paprika (10 g)
Cumin (10 g)
Chili powder (10.4 g)
Italian seasoning (8 g)
Poultry seasoning (6 g)
Montreal (steak) seasoning (8.3 g)
Black pepper (8 g)
Cayenne pepper (7.2 g)
Fennel seeds (8 g)
Oregano, fresh (5.2 g) or dried (4 g)
Curry powder (8 g)

RECOMMENDED DRY BASE INGREDIENTS (1 cup)

Buckwheat flour (120 g)
Unsweetened protein powder (128 g)
Bread crumbs (115 g)
Cornmeal (140 g)
Oatmeal (80 g)

RECOMMENDED TEXTURE INGREDIENTS (½ cup)

Finely chopped walnuts (60 g)
Chopped olives (50 g)
Avocado cubes (73 g)
Sundried tomatoes (not oil packed) (28 g)

Leftover cooked rice, quinoa, or other grain or pseudograin (165 to 185 g)
Fresh parsley, cilantro, or basil (20 to 30 g)

EXAMPLE: CLASSIC SLIDERS

1 can (15½ ounces, or 440 g) or 1½ cups (258 g) cooked black beans, drained and rinsed
½ cup (80 g) chopped onion
1 clove garlic, minced
1 cup (70 g) mushrooms, rough-chopped
½ cup (50 g) celery, rough-chopped
½ cup (75 g) green pepper, rough-chopped
1 tablespoon (15 g) ketchup

1 tablespoon (11 g) mustard
1 teaspoon liquid smoke
2 teaspoons soy sauce or vegan Worcestershire sauce
3 teaspoons (6 g) Montreal steak seasoning
1 teaspoon Italian seasoning
1 cup (115 g) panko bread crumbs
½ cup (60 g) walnuts, finely chopped

Follow recipe directions for The Incredible Veggie Burger Formula on page 135 using those ingredients.

YIELD: ABOUT 18 SMALL PATTIES (5-6 DINNER-SIZED SERVINGS)

PER PATTY: 72 Calories; 2 g Fat (27.3% calories from fat); 4 g Protein; 10 g Carbohydrate; 3 g Dietary Fiber; trace Cholesterol; 257 mg Sodium

EASY HOMEMADE PIZZA

A lot of people are intimidated by the idea of making pizza themselves. I imagine they picture several hours of mixing and kneading dough and every surface of the kitchen covered with flour. Fortunately, this food processor pizza dough recipe makes it fast and easy. You've still got to let the dough rise for an hour, but the actual hands-on time is less than 10 minutes, and you end up with a healthy, homemade pizza.

FOR THE DOUGH:

2¼ teaspoons (9 g or 1 packet)
   instant yeast
1 cup (235 ml) lukewarm water
1½ cups (180 g) whole wheat flour
1 cup (137 g) bread flour
1 teaspoon salt
2 teaspoons sugar
1 tablespoon (15 ml) olive oil

FOR THE PIZZAS:

1½ cups (368 g) Tasty Three-Ingredient
   Tomato Sauce (page 144), divided
1 tablespoon (6 g) Italian seasoning
1 teaspoon garlic powder
1 cup (260 g) Cashew "Cheese" Spread
   and Sauce (page 145) or (112 g) Daiya
   mozzarella-style vegan cheese

To make the dough: Stir the yeast into the water and let stand 5 minutes.

Meanwhile, put the flours, salt, and sugar in a food processor. Pulse once or twice to mix. Turn on the food processor and slowly add the yeast mixture and the oil. Within a few seconds, the dough should come together in a ball.

The dough should be smooth and slightly tacky, but not wet and sticky.

If it's sticky, add more flour, a tablespoon (11 g) at a time, and process. If it's dry or not coming together, add more water, a tablespoon (15 ml) at a time, and process for up to a minute.

Turn the dough out onto a floured surface, knead it for just a second, and then cut it in half.

For each piece of dough, grab both ends of the cut side and bring them together, pinching to seal so that the cut side is no longer exposed. Place each piece in its own, lightly oiled, large bowl, cover with a damp kitchen towel, and let rise for an hour, so that it roughly doubles in size. If the dough doesn't rise enough, let it sit a bit longer.

Punch the risen dough balls down and one at a time, use a rolling pin to roll out on a lightly floured surface so that they're each 12 to 14 inches (30 to 35 cm) round and about ¼ inch (6 mm) thick.

To make the pizzas: If you have a pizza stone, position a rack near the bottom of your oven and place the stone on it and position another rack several inches above it. The purpose of using the stone is to get a nice, crispy bottom of the crust. You only move the pizza to the stone during the last 2 to 3 minutes of cooking; otherwise, the bottom burns. In this step, we are preheating the stone, but you need to have another rack where the pizza will cook until it's time to move to the stone. Preheat the oven to 450°F (230°C, or gas mark 8). If you're using a stone, allow about an hour of preheat time.

Place your rolled dough onto a lightly oiled pizza screen or baking sheet. Top each pizza with about a half cup (115 g) of sauce and spread it around in an even layer. Sprinkle with Italian seasoning, garlic powder, and any other seasoning you like.

If using Cashew "Cheese" Spread and Sauce, put it on after the pizzas are almost finished baking (see below). If using Daiya cheese, sprinkle it on now.

Place the baking sheet or pizza screen with the pizzas on the top rack of the oven. Bake for 8 to 10 minutes until the crust is golden brown and looks about a minute or two from being done.

If using Cashew "Cheese" Spread and Sauce, remove the pizzas from the oven and then drizzle some of the sauce on top. Lightly spread it around with a knife or spoon or leave it in dollops, margherita-style. If you are using a pizza stone, place the pizzas directly on the stone. If you're not using the Cashew "Cheese" Spread and Sauce, just leave your pizza in the oven for another minute or two until it's done.

Return the pizzas to the oven. Bake for another two or three minutes until the crust is crisp on the bottom and completely done on top. If the cheesy sauce isn't warm, put the pizza under the broiler for a few seconds to heat it up.

YIELD: 2 MEDIUM-SIZED PIZZAS, ENOUGH TO SERVE ABOUT 4

PER SERVING: 580 Calories; 27 g Fat (39.4% calories from fat); 17 g Protein; 75 g Carbohydrate; 9 g Dietary Fiber; 0 mg Cholesterol; 1221 mg Sodium

RECIPE NOTE

Although the Cashew "Cheese" Spread and Sauce is the healthier option, Daiya cheese will produce a more traditional pizza. For the cashew sauce, you'll need to have soaked the cashews for at least four hours, so plan ahead.

COWBOY CHILI

If you're not up for making the coffee called for in this recipe, you can substitute more vegetable broth. If you are, decaf will also work just fine. (I'd probably skip the hazelnut flavor though.) Although brown rice or bulgur wheat is the serving suggestion, try pasta, too—you can sprinkle in a little cinnamon and call it Cincinnati-style. Our toddler would never eat chili alone, but mixed with pasta and called chili mac, it's a hit!

1 tablespoon (15 ml) olive or grapeseed oil
1 small onion, chopped
1 green bell pepper, chopped
1 cup (150 g) canned hominy
2 cups (134 g) packed collard greens, chopped
2 cloves garlic, minced
1/2 teaspoon salt
1 tablespoon (7.5 g) chili powder
2 teaspoons cumin
1 1/2 teaspoons smoked paprika
1/2 teaspoon oregano
1 can (28 ounces, or 795 g) stewed tomatoes

1 cup (235 ml) vegetable broth
1/2 cup (120 ml) brewed coffee
1 tablespoon (15 ml) hot sauce or other pepper sauce, more for serving
1 can (15 1/2 ounces, or 440 g) black-eyed peas, drained and rinsed
1 can (15 1/2 ounces, or 440 g) kidney beans, drained and rinsed
6 to 8 cups (1.2 to 1.6 Kg) cooked brown rice or (1.1 to 1.5 Kg) bulgur wheat, for serving
Lime juice, for serving
Cashew "Cheese" Spread (page 145) or sliced avocado, for serving (optional)

Heat the oil in a large pot over medium heat. Add the onion, bell pepper, hominy, and collard greens and cook, stirring frequently, for about 7 minutes or until onion is lightly browned.

Add the garlic, salt, chili powder, cumin, paprika, and oregano and cook for an additional minute. Add the tomatoes, vegetable broth, coffee, and hot sauce and then stir in the beans.

Bring to a boil. Reduce the heat to medium and simmer, covered, for at least 25 minutes. The longer you cook the chili and the lower the temperature, the more the flavors will meld and the better the chili will taste.

Adjust the salt and seasonings to taste and serve over cooked brown rice or bulgur wheat, with more hot sauce, lime juice, and Cashew "Cheese" spread or sliced avocado for garnish.

YIELD: 8 SERVINGS

PER SERVING: 764 Calories; 16 g Fat (18.7% calories from fat); 36 g Protein; 124 g Carbohydrate; 26 g Dietary Fiber; trace Cholesterol; 770 mg Sodium

THAI PINEAPPLE COCONUT CURRY WITH BOK CHOY AND TOFU

I often make Thai curries using Fine Cooking's "Create Your Own" recipe generator (www.finecooking.com/articles/cyor/thai-curry.aspx), choosing what vegetables I'm in the mood for or have at home. This recipe isn't exactly what you'll get from there, as I always end up using more vegetables than they suggest and have to substitute for the fish sauce, but it's close. The next time you're in the mood for Thai, give it a try!

1 can (13½ ounces or 400 ml) light coconut milk, shaken and divided

¼ cup (64 g) red curry paste

1 tablespoon (6 g) fresh ginger, minced

1 cup (235 ml) vegetable broth

2 tablespoons (30 g) light brown sugar

2 teaspoons miso paste

4 teaspoons (20 ml) tamari or soy sauce, plus more to taste

2 large carrots, sliced ⅛ inch (3 mm) thick

4 sticks of dried or fresh lemongrass, 2 inches (5 cm) long

1 pound (455 g) extra-firm tofu, drained and cubed

4 baby bok choy stalks, chopped into 1 inch (2.5 cm) lengths, leaves roughly chopped and reserved

1 cup (165 g) bite-size pineapple chunks

¾ cup (30 g or 1 bunch) loosely packed fresh basil, roughly chopped

Lime wedges, for garnish

Sriracha sauce, for serving

Add ½ cup (120 ml) coconut milk to a large pot or Dutch oven over medium heat and simmer until it reduces by half, about 5 minutes. Whisk in the curry paste, add the ginger, and cook for 1 minute. Then stir in the broth, sugar, miso, tamari or soy sauce, and remaining coconut milk. Bring to a simmer over medium-high heat.

Add the carrots and lemongrass and simmer for 2 minutes. Then add the tofu and simmer for 2 more minutes. Finally, add the bok choy (stalks only) and pineapple and simmer until everything is tender, another minute or so.

Remove the pot from the heat. Season to taste with more tamari or soy sauce and stir in the reserved bok choy leaves and basil. Serve with lime wedges, sriracha, and more tamari or soy sauce.

Important: Remove the lemongrass pieces before serving, so nobody chokes!

YIELD: 4 SERVINGS

PER SERVING: 449 Calories; 22 g Fat (41.6% calories from fat); 20 g Protein; 51 g Carbohydrate; 5 g Dietary Fiber; 3 mg Cholesterol; 1599 mg Sodium

SUPER SIDES, SNACKS, AND SAUCES

THE BEST DAMN CHEEZE DIP I EVER ATE

My friend Brad has a punk-rock style vegan cookzine called Please Don't Feed the Bears, *and one of the most popular recipes is for this delicious "cheese" sauce. Liquid smoke adds depth, and arrowroot makes this nacho cheese-style sauce nice and creamy. This dip solidifies somewhat when you store it in the refrigerator; to bring it back to its cheese-dip consistency, add a little water and reheat on the stovetop or microwave. –Matthew Ruscigno*

2 cups (475 ml) water
¹/₃ cup (32 g) nutritional yeast
¹/₄ cup (60 g) tahini
¹/₄ cup (32 g) arrowroot powder or
    7 teaspoons (19 g) corn starch
2 tablespoons (28 ml) lemon juice

1 tablespoon (6.9 g) onion powder
1 teaspoon salt
2 dashes liquid smoke
2 tablespoons (19 g) bell peppers, diced
2 jalapeño peppers, minced (the bottled
    ones work great here)

Combine everything in a blender except the bell and jalapeño peppers and blend. Pour the mixture into a pot, add the peppers, and whisk rapidly over high heat until mixture thickens.

This should only take a few minutes, so be careful not to let the mixture stick!

YIELD: 2¹/₂ CUPS (625 G)

TOTAL RECIPE: 681 Calories; 38 g Fat (45.4% calories from fat); 37 g Protein; 65 g Carbohydrate; 25 g Dietary Fiber; trace Cholesterol; 2456 mg Sodium

S'NUTS

S'nuts are super, sexy, smoky, snacking nuts. At Plant, we serve S'nuts during dinner service as a pre-dinner snack. The only difference between the recipe here and those that we serve for amuse bouche *is that we smoke our snacking nuts over apple or cherry wood for about 5 minutes. If you have a smoker, then doing so will take your S'nuts to another level. —Jason Sellers, chef and co-owner at Plant restaurant, Asheville, North Carolina*

4 cups (380 to 540 g) of your favorite energy-rich nuts (e.g., hazelnuts, almonds, cashew, pecans)
2 tablespoons (40 g) maple syrup

1 teaspoon sea salt
Large pinch each black pepper and onion powder

Preheat the oven to 350° (180°C or gas mark 4). Combine the nuts and the maple syrup in a mixing bowl and stir with a rubber spatula until the nuts are coated. Then season with salt, pepper, and onion powder and stir again to make uniform. Spread the nuts out in a single layer on a baking pan covered with parchment paper or a reusable baking sheet. Bake for 12 to 15 minutes until lightly browned. Cool and store or mix with fruit and seeds for a nutritive trail mix.

YIELD: 4 CUPS (ABOUT 450 G, DEPENDING ON NUTS USED)

PER SERVING: 2342 Calories; 198 G Fat (71.3% Calories from fat); 76 G Protein; 104 G Carbohydrate; 41 G Dietary Fiber; 0 Mg Cholesterol; 1925 Mg Sodium

TASTY THREE-INGREDIENT TOMATO SAUCE

The simplicity of this tomato sauce is part of its delicious appeal. Because it has only three ingredients, it's versatile enough to be used in a variety of recipes. Best of all, it takes just about no active time and only 20 minutes of simmering before it's ready. I recommend making a large batch and freezing the sauce in cup-size portions so that you can pull them out for use in various recipes.

1 can (28 ounces, or 785 g) whole peeled tomatoes

¼ cup (60 ml) olive oil (optional)

½ teaspoon sea salt

Lightly pulse the entire contents of the can of tomatoes in a blender or food processor to your desired consistency. (I like to leave a few chunks.) If you don't have a blender or processor, you can do this with a potato masher.

Heat the oil in a large saucepan over medium heat. If you want more flavors in your tomato sauce, such as garlic, crushed red pepper, or herbs, add them now and cook for a minute or so before you add the tomatoes.

Add the tomatoes, lower the heat to medium-low, and let the sauce simmer uncovered, stirring occasionally, until it thickens, about 20 minutes.

YIELD: 2 CUPS (490 g)

TOTAL RECIPE: 635 Calories; 56 g Fat (74.9% calories from fat); 7 g Protein; 35 g Carbohydrate; 8 g Dietary Fiber; 0 mg Cholesterol; 2115 mg Sodium

CASHEW "CHEESE" SPREAD AND SAUCE

This cashew "cheese" works just about anywhere regular cheese does, and it's so much better for you. On its own or with a few seasonings, it works as a spread for crostini or a dip for vegetables, and by adding water, you can use it to drizzle as a garnish or even as a cheese sauce for pizza. Props to Dreena Burton and her amazing cookbook Let Them Eat Vegan *for first inspiring me to start making and using cashew cheese.*

2 cups (280 g) raw cashews, soaked 4 to 6 hours in water, drained and rinsed

2 tablespoons (28 ml) lemon juice

1 small clove garlic

$\frac{1}{2}$ teaspoon sea salt

For the spread: $\frac{1}{4}$ cup (60 ml) water, plus more for thinning *or*

For the sauce: $\frac{1}{2}$ cup (120 ml) water, plus more for thinning

Combine all the ingredients in a food processor; process for several minutes until completely smooth. Add extra water and continue to process until you achieve the desired consistency for either a spread or sauce.

YIELD: ABOUT 2 CUPS (500 G) OF SPREAD, OR 2$\frac{1}{4}$ CUPS (563 G) SAUCE

TOTAL RECIPE: 1088 Calories; 89 g Fat (69.0% calories from fat); 35 g Protein; 55 g Carbohydrate; 6 g Dietary Fiber; 0 mg Cholesterol; 2280 mg Sodium

SIMPLE INDIAN STREET BREAD

It's tough to find vegan versions of the Indian breads naan and roti in most stores, so here's an easy Indian bread recipe that can be made at home, with almost no work! Use whatever proportions of whole wheat flour and white flour you like; the more whole wheat you use, the healthier, but without any white flour, these breads turn out a bit too dense.

1 cup (125 g) flour, a blend of whole
   wheat and white

½ teaspoon salt

About ¾ cup (175 ml) cold water

2 to 3 teaspoons (10 to 15 ml)
   grapeseed oil

Mix the flour and salt in a large bowl and then gradually add the water and incorporate it into the flour with your fingers until a firm dough comes together. When it does, knead it in your hands for a few minutes—you want it to be just slightly tacky, but not sticky. If it's too sticky, add more flour; if it's too dry, add more water. Place the dough back in the bowl and cover with a damp kitchen towel for an hour.

On a lightly floured surface, separate the dough into 8 small balls and use a rolling pin to roll each out to about ⅛ inch (3 mm) thick disks. Heat a large skillet over medium heat and working in batches, brush the sides of each disk with the oil and cook for about a minute per side until brown in a few spots.

YIELD: 8 SMALL BREADS

PER SERVING: 67 Calories; 1 g Fat (17.6% calories from fat); 2 g Protein; 12 g Carbohydrate; trace Dietary Fiber; 0 mg Cholesterol; 134 mg Sodium

SERVING SUGGESTIONS

These breads are nice alternatives to rice for serving alongside Indian dishes—we often use them to scoop White Bean Coconut Curry (page 122), Plant Restaurant's Curried Lentils (page 127), or Super Quick Red Lentils and Rice (page 126) right from a bowl (fork or spoon optional!).

Please cut to fit.

PERFECT PEANUT SAUCE

Peanut sauce is so delicious that every time I make it, I can't believe how easy it is. This recipe is "lazy-fancy" and so much better than anything you'd buy in a bottle. And way cheaper. Peanuts are magical legumes that have an unbelievable number of uses. Also, it's easy to adjust the spiciness, sweetness, and thickness of this dish, as well as the amount of garlic, depending on your mood. It's super fun to make, and it's easy! —Matthew Ruscigno

½ cup (130 g) peanut butter

½ cup (120 ml) vegetable broth

1 tablespoon (15 ml) soy sauce, more to taste

1 teaspoon rice vinegar (or other mild vinegar)

1 tablespoon sweetener (agave nectar [20 g], maple syrup [20 g], unrefined sugar [13 g], etc.)

2 to 4 cloves garlic, to taste

1 thumb-sized piece of fresh ginger, peeled and diced

Sriracha hot sauce, to taste

Put all ingredients in a blender and blend. Taste and then add more soy sauce, garlic, sweeter, or broth to suit your mood.

YIELD: ABOUT FOUR ¼-CUP (60 G) SERVINGS

PER SERVING: 230 Calories; 17 g Fat (62.6% calories from fat); 9 g Protein; 14 g Carbohydrate; 3 g Dietary Fiber; trace Cholesterol; 619 mg Sodium

SERVING SUGGESTIONS

Serve this sauce over sautéed vegetables (my favorites are broccoli and red bell peppers), rice, or noodles. It keeps well in the fridge, so I make a huge amount and eat it for a few days. I'll even dip raw vegetables into it while it's cold. Yum!

DINOSAUR KALE CHIPS

The way some people rave about kale chips, you'd think they're even better than potato chips. I'm not going to go that far, but they've got a taste all their own and a crispness that satisfies that snack-food urge while still providing a lot of nutrition. You can retain more of kale's nutrition in your chips by cooking it at a very low temperature for a longer period of time, but I've found that 300°F (150°C or gas mark 2) results in the best texture, so that's what I call for here.

9 ounces (255 g or about 6 cups) kale (I like Lacinato, also called dinosaur kale)

2 teaspoons olive oil or melted coconut oil

½ teaspoon sea salt

½ teaspoon nutritional yeast

Zest of 1 lemon (optional)

Preheat the oven to 300°F (150°C, or gas mark 2).

Tear or cut the kale leaves away from their thick stems, discard the stems, and then tear or roughly chop the leaves into bite-size pieces. Add the oil to a large bowl, toss the kale leaves to coat, and then lay the leaves out on a baking sheet so that they do not overlap (this is important for getting them to cook evenly). You may need to use two baking sheets or work in batches to accommodate the entire bunch of kale.

Sprinkle with sea salt, nutritional yeast, and lemon zest, if using.

Bake for about 10 to 15 minutes until the kale chips are lightly crisped. As ovens vary, you'll need to pay close attention the first time you make these to determine exactly how long to cook them—you don't want to let them burn.

YIELD: 3 LOOSELY PACKED CUPS (90 G)

TOTAL RECIPE: 213 Calories; 11 g Fat (40.8% calories from fat); 9 g Protein; 26 g Carbohydrate; 6 g Dietary Fiber; 0 mg Cholesterol; 1051 mg Sodium

GRILL-SMOKED EGGPLANT DIP

Smoked eggplant is the backbone of several delicious dishes, including the Indian baingan barta *and the Middle-Eastern* baba ganoush. *This recipe is essentially the latter, but it's so different from any other version I've tested that I'm hesitant to call it by its proper name. Whatever you call this eggplant dip, it's wonderful and a nice change from hummus. The skin of the eggplants will char on the grill, imparting an incredible smoky flavor that, balanced by the lemon juice, makes for a sublime dip for pitas or vegetables.*

2 globe eggplants (about 2 pounds [910 g] total)
6 tablespoons (90 ml) olive oil

Juice of 1 lemon, more to taste
2 teaspoons (12 g) salt, more to taste

First, smoke the eggplants: Crank your outdoor grill up to 600°F (315°C) or as close as you can get to that.

Pierce the eggplants all over with a fork and put them on the grill (smoke more eggplants at the same time if you want to use the flesh for other dishes). Close the grill. Use tongs to rotate the eggplants every 10 to 15 minutes and cook for as little as half an hour and up to a full hour. The longer you leave them on there, the smokier the eggplant will get. You want the flesh to be nice and soft but the skins to get charred and crisp. Remove the eggplants from the grill and allow to cool. Carefully cut the eggplants in half lengthwise. Scoop out the flesh (seeds are fine, too) with a spoon and set aside, discarding the brittle skins. (Others will tell you to peel the skins off, but that leaves lots of char behind, so I prefer to scoop.)

To make the dip: Place the eggplant flesh in a food processor and with the motor running, stream in the oil. Add the lemon juice and salt, pulse a few times, and then add more lemon juice and salt to taste.

Serve as a dip for vegetables or pitas.

YIELD: 1 CUP (230 G)

TOTAL RECIPE: 1206 Calories; 84 g Fat (58.1% calories from fat); 19 g Protein; 118 g Carbohydrate; 47 g Dietary Fiber; 0 mg Cholesterol; 4320 mg Sodium

LEMON GARLIC HUMMUS (WITH JALAPEÑO VARIATION)

If you're new to a plant-based diet, let me give you a little more advice: learn to love your hummus. It's such a hearty, healthy snack, not just when nothing else is available, but anytime. Dip vegetables in it, spread it on crackers with some olives, or fill up a pita with it. We make sandwiches with sprouted-grain bread, whatever vegetables we have on hand, and hummus and bring them on long car trips. The sandwiches are one of my toddler's favorite foods! Note: If you're going to use the liquid from the chickpea can instead of oil, reduce the amount of garlic to one clove and skip the step of cooking it.

3 tablespoons (45 ml) olive oil (or 3 tablespoons [45 ml] reserved liquid from chickpea can)

3 cloves garlic, roughly chopped

1 can (15½ ounces, or 440 g) or 1½ cups (246 g) cooked chickpeas, drained and rinsed

1 tablespoon (15 g) tahini

2 tablespoons (28 ml) lemon juice, more to taste

1 tablespoon (15 ml) tamari or soy sauce, more to taste

1 small jalapeño pepper, seeded and minced (remove ribs for less heat), optional

Heat the oil in a small saucepan over medium heat. Add the garlic and cook, stirring frequently so that it cooks evenly, for 3 or 4 minutes. Avoid burning the garlic, but allow it to get a little color, as it adds a deeper flavor. Remove from the heat and allow to cool.

Add the chickpeas, tahini, lemon juice, tamari or soy sauce, and jalapeño (if using) to a food processor and pulse a few times to combine. Scrape down the sides with a spatula and then, with the motor running, slowly pour in the oil and garlic from the saucepan (avoid using the feed tube on the food processor because the garlic will clog the narrow opening).

Scrape down the sides of the food processor once more if necessary and continue to process. If the hummus is too thick, add a little bit of water, 1 tablespoon (15 ml) at time, until the desired consistency is reached.

Taste and add more lemon juice and tamari or soy sauce, to taste, pulsing a few times to incorporate before serving.

YIELD: ABOUT 1½ CUPS (375 G)

TOTAL RECIPE: 1204 Calories; 60 g Fat (43.5% calories from fat); 44 g Protein; 131 g Carbohydrate; 17 g Dietary Fiber; 0 mg Cholesterol; 1056 mg Sodium

BLACK BEAN HUMMUS

It's funny how completely different hummus tastes when you replace just one ingredient—all of a sudden it seems like a perfect match for corn chips instead of pitas. And because corn chips are generally saltier than pitas, this recipe calls for slightly less salt than the other hummus recipes in this book. Note: If you're going to use the liquid from the black bean can instead of oil, reduce the amount of garlic to one clove and skip the step of cooking it.

3 tablespoons (45 ml) olive oil (or 3 tablespoons [45 ml] reserved liquid from a can of black beans)

3 cloves garlic, roughly chopped

1 can (15¹/₂ ounces, or 440 g) or 1¹/₂ cups (258 g) cooked black beans, drained and rinsed

1 tablespoon (15 g) tahini

2 tablespoons (28 ml) lemon juice, more to taste

¹/₄ teaspoon salt

¹/₂ teaspoon ground cumin

Heat the oil in a small saucepan over medium heat. Add the garlic and cook, stirring frequently so that it cooks evenly, for 3 or 4 minutes. Avoid burning the garlic, but let it get a little color, as it adds a deeper flavor to the hummus. Remove from the heat and cool.

Add the black beans, tahini, lemon juice, salt, and cumin to a food processor and pulse a few times to combine.

Scrape down the sides with a spatula and then, with the motor running, slowly pour in the oil and garlic from the saucepan (don't use the feed tube on the food processor because the garlic pieces will clog the narrow opening).

Scrape down the sides once more if necessary and continue to process—the longer you let the machine run, the smoother your hummus will be. If the hummus is too thick, add a little bit of water, 1 tablespoon (15 ml) at time, until the desired consistency is reached.

Add more lemon juice and salt, to taste, pulsing a few times to incorporate, before serving

---

YIELD: ABOUT 1¹/₂ CUPS (375 G)

TOTAL RECIPE: 1052 Calories; 51 g Fat (42.5% calories from fat); 42 g Protein; 113 g Carbohydrate; 40 g Dietary Fiber; 0 mg Cholesterol; 559 mg Sodium

BUFFALO HUMMUS

Of all the foods I missed when I went vegetarian, buffalo chicken was number one. It wasn't so much the chicken I craved as the tangy, burn-your-lips spiciness of buffalo sauce. For a while, I just bought bottles of it and put it on anything and everything, but because most buffalo sauce is made with butter, that stopped working once I went vegan. Fortunately, my sister Christine came up with this variation, which combines my favorite flavor with one of the foods I eat most often (hummus). Booyah. As with the other hummus recipes, substitute the liquid from the can of chickpeas if you want to avoid oil.

1 can (15¹/₂ ounces, or 440 g) or 1¹/₂ cups (246 g) cooked chickpeas, drained and rinsed
¹/₂ teaspoon cumin
¹/₂ teaspoon smoked paprika
¹/₄ teaspoon salt
2 cloves garlic
2 tablespoons (30 g) tahini

1 tablespoon (15 ml) hot sauce
1 tablespoon (15 ml) lemon juice
¹/₂ cup (90 g) jarred roasted red pepper
2 tablespoons (28 ml) olive oil (or substitute 2 tablespoons [28 ml] liquid from chickpea can)
Cayenne pepper, to taste, for serving

Combine all the ingredients except the oil and cayenne in a food processor. Pulse a few times to combine and then scrape down the sides. With the motor running, stream in the oil through the feed tube.

Continue to run the motor until you reach the desired consistency; I like to let it go for 5 or more minutes to get it really smooth.

Add more salt, lemon juice, and hot sauce, to taste, and then sprinkle with cayenne pepper before serving.

YIELD: 2 CUPS (500 G)

TOTAL RECIPE: 1173 Calories; 55 g Fat (40.8% calories from fat); 45 g Protein; 135 g Carbohydrate; 20 g Dietary Fiber; 0 mg Cholesterol; 976 mg Sodium

ROASTED BRUSSELS SPROUTS

Brussels sprouts pack a lot of nutrition into a tiny package, from vitamins C and K to potassium and manganese. At my restaurant, Plant, we only roast them. Roasting makes for the perfect texture and flavor, intensifies their beautiful shades of green, and maintains much of their amino acid profile. Here, nutritional yeast pairs well with the natural bitterness of the sprouts and boosts B-vitamin levels. For a quick leftover dish, roast enough for two or three meals; they will keep covered in the refrigerator for a couple of days. Just add a little bit of stock or broth and reheat in a pan. —Jason Sellers, chef and co-owner of Plant restaurant, Asheville, North Carolina

8 cups (704 g) Brussels sprouts, stems trimmed, and cut in half if larger than 1 inch (2.5 cm) in diameter

3 tablespoons (45 ml) good-quality olive or safflower oil

2 tablespoons (12 g) nutritional yeast

Salt and black pepper, to taste

Preheat the oven to 400° (200° C or gas mark 6). Toss the Brussels sprouts gently with the oil in a large mixing bowl. Season with the nutritional yeast, salt, and pepper and spread out in a single layer on a baking tray. Leave room between the sprouts so that the air can circulate and lightly caramelize the leaves. Roast 8 to 10 minutes or until tender and brown peaks are visible. Avoid overcooking, as the sprouts will become mushy.

YIELD: 8 CUPS (704 G)

TOTAL RECIPE: 728 Calories; 43 g Fat (48.4% calories from fat); 33 g Protein; 71 g Carbohydrate, 33 g Dietary Fiber; 0 mg Cholesterol; 186 mg Sodium

SNEAKY-HEALTHY DESSERTS

BLACK BEAN BROWNIES

Of all the recipes on my blog, this one from my sister Christine is arguably the most popular. Black beans in brownies sound weird, I know, but you absolutely can't taste them. The result is a delicious dessert you can feel good about eating—and sharing, as most people won't even detect that anything is different from regular brownies!

FOR THE DRY INGREDIENTS:

1½ cups (180 g) whole wheat flour
1 teaspoon salt
1 teaspoon baking powder
2¼ cups (450 g) raw sugar
1¼ cups (113 g) cocoa powder
4 teaspoons (4 g) instant coffee powder
1½ cups (173 g) chopped hazelnuts

FOR THE WET INGREDIENTS:

1 can (15½ ounces, or 440 g) black beans
1 teaspoon vanilla extract
1 cup (235 ml) water

Preheat the oven to 350°F (180°C, or gas mark 4).

Add the dry ingredients to a large mixing bowl and stir to combine.

Drain and rinse the beans thoroughly and then rinse out any remaining liquid inside the can. Return the beans back to the can and fill with water. Then dump the contents of the can (beans and water) into a food processor or blender to purée. Add the purée to the dry ingredients, along with the vanilla extract and 1 cup (235 ml) water. Stir to combine.

Pour the batter into a greased 9 x 13-inch pan (23 x 33 cm). Bake for 25 to 30 minutes, rotating the pan about halfway through.

When the brownies are finished, they should be firm in the center and the edges will be slightly puffy and starting to pull away from the sides. Avoid overbaking them because they will keep baking once you take them out.

Let brownies cool completely and cut into 24 squares (a 2 inch [5 cm] square cookie cutter works well here).

YIELD: 24 BROWNIES

PER SERVING: 217 Calories; 6 g Fat (21.2% calories from fat); 7 g Protein; 39 g Carbohydrate; 6 g Dietary Fiber; 0 mg Cholesterol; 112 mg Sodium

CHOCOLATE AVOCADO MOUSSE

This is my genius sister Christine's totally guiltless version of chocolate mousse. Most of the fat comes from the avocados and peanut butter. And don't worry, it looks like regular chocolate mousse—not green, I promise. And you'd never guess from the rich taste that there's anything healthy in there.

4 ounces (115 g) semisweet, dairy-free chocolate

1 tablespoon (14 g) coconut oil

2 avocados, peeled and pitted

2 tablespoons (10 g) cocoa powder

¼ cup (80 g) pure maple syrup

2 teaspoons vanilla extract

Pinch of salt

¼ cup (64 g) natural peanut butter

Put the oil in a microwave-safe bowl, add the chocolate, and stir to coat. Microwave for 45 seconds. Stir and then microwave for 30 more seconds. Repeat with decreasing times until the chocolate is melted and smooth.

In a separate bowl, mash the avocado roughly with a fork or pastry cutter and then whisk to get the lumps out. You can use a food processor if you'd like, but a hand whisk works fine and burns a few calories!

Combine the melted chocolate with the smooth avocado. Add the remaining ingredients except for the peanut butter. (Tip: Measure the syrup with the same spoon you used for the oil so that it slides right out.)

Use a spatula to force the mixture through a fine mesh strainer to get any last lumps out and then mix in the peanut butter.

Divide among four bowls. Top with sprinkles, fruit, or anything your heart desires and dig in.

YIELD: 4 SERVINGS

PER SERVING: 511 Calories; 35 g Fat (59.6% calories from fat); 8 g Protein; 45 g Carbohydrate; 6 g Dietary Fiber; 0 mg Cholesterol; 106 mg Sodium

RECIPE NOTES

If you don't like microwaving food, use a double boiler to melt the chocolate in the oil without scorching it or a makeshift one using a heatproof bowl over a slowly simmering pot of water.

SWEET POTATO PIE PARFAIT

Sweet potatoes are a high-fiber, nutritionally dense carb and ideal for a pre-workout snack. These parfaits are a great way to satisfy your sweet tooth with something a little fancy and decadent that won't put you too far off track. —Sara Beth Russert, *vegan baker and bodybuilder, recently named National Donut Champion on* The Food Network Challenge *for her vegan donuts*

FOR THE PUDDING:

2 medium sweet potatoes
   (about 16 ounces [455 g] in weight)
½ block (about 6 ounces [170 g]) firm
   tofu, drained and rinsed
1 tablespoon (7 g) cinnamon
¼ teaspoon ground ginger
⅛ teaspoon nutmeg
2 teaspoons alcohol-free vanilla extract
   or pulp from 1 vanilla bean
Pinch of salt
1 to 2 teaspoons sweetener, such as agave
   nectar, to taste (optional)

FOR THE TOPPING:

¼ cup (20 g) gluten-free old-fashioned
   rolled oats (not instant)
2 tablespoons (13 g) chopped almonds
2 tablespoons (16 g) cacao nibs
2 dates, soaked in water for 20 minutes,
   pitted, and chopped
Pinch of salt

Preheat oven to 400°F (200°C or gas mark 6). Bake the sweet potatoes on a baking sheet for 45 minutes to an hour. Remove from oven and allow to cool for at least 30 minutes.

To make the pudding: If using a high-speed blender, you can leave the sweet potato skins on, otherwise remove them. Combine sweet potatoes with the rest of the pudding ingredients, except the sweetener, in a blender or food processor and purée until completely smooth. Add the sweetener to taste. Chill the pudding until it is completely cool.

To make the topping: Combine all the topping ingredients in a sauté pan and toast over medium heat until the oats begin to brown, about 3 to 5 minutes. Stir frequently so nothing burns. Allow the topping to cool.

To assemble, put a heaping half cup (123 g) of pudding into a small dish or to be extra fancy, use glasses. Top each serving with one-fifth of the topping.

YIELD: Approximately 5 servings, and definitely counts as a meal on its own!

PER SERVING: 150 Calories; 5 g Fat (30.9% calories from fat); 4 g Protein; 23 g Carbohydrate; 5 g Dietary Fiber; 0 mg Cholesterol; 62 mg Sodium

OATMEAL FLAX SPELT COOKIES

What!? A dessert recipe without beans in it? It's true, but these wonderful oatmeal cookies are made with flaxseeds and spelt flour, an ancient form of wheat (feel free to substitute whole wheat if you can't find spelt).

1³/₄ cups (210 g) spelt flour
1¹/₂ cups (120 g) oats
1¹/₂ teaspoons baking soda
³/₄ teaspoon salt
³/₄ cup (168 g) coconut oil
¹/₂ cup (115 g) brown sugar

¹/₂ cup (100 g) unrefined sugar
1¹/₂ cups (168 g) ground flaxseed
¹/₄ cup (60 g) applesauce
1 teaspoon vanilla extract
1 cup (150 g) dried currants or
  other fruit

Preheat the oven to 350°F (180°C or gas mark 4).

Mix together the spelt flour, oats, baking soda, and salt. Set aside.

Beat the coconut oil with a whisk until smooth. You may have to microwave it to soften it a bit. Whisk in the sugars and then stir in the flaxseed. Add the applesauce and vanilla extract and mix until uniform.

Stir the dry ingredients into the wet. Fold in the currants.

Using an ice cream scoop, place large mounds of cookie dough on a greased cookie sheet. Flatten the cookies with your palm so they are about 3 inches (7.5 cm) across.

Bake for 16 minutes, turning the pan around about halfway through baking.

YIELD: 15 LARGE, BAKERY-STYLE COOKIES

PER SERVING: 255 Calories; 15 g Fat (43.7% calories from fat); 5 g Protein; 40 g Carbohydrate; 5 g Dietary Fiber; 0 mg Cholesterol; 239 mg Sodium

RUNNING ON PLANTS

CHAPTER 6

HOW YOU CAN LEARN TO LOVE RUNNING

I have a theory about why so many people tell themselves that they don't like running. Remember how we all used to have to do the mile run in gym class? One day, instead of playing dodge ball, floor hockey, or something else that was fun, our gym teachers would make us run as fast as we could for a whole mile.

For most of us, it was the only time we'd run that far all year. Our times were recorded, and if you were the ten-minute miler in the class or simply the slowest, you were laughed at.

In this way, we learned to run. Go as hard as you can for a mile. It'll hurt, you'll probably cough a lot, and that last lap and sprint to the finish line will be pure pain. But in a few minutes, that miserable mile will be done, and you won't have to do it again until next year.

If this is running, is it any wonder so many of us say we hate it?

Before I was a runner, that's exactly what running meant to me, but I'd run in-between weightlifting sessions anyway, hoping to burn some fat. I remember the first time I ever pushed the distance to two miles on the treadmill—as fast as I could manage, of course—and I found it so painful and boring that I distinctly recall thinking, "If this is how it feels to be a runner, there's no way I'll ever become one."

If this sounds familiar, take heart. I am living proof that the ability to run well isn't something you're either born with or you're not, though there's no denying that some people have a gift for running. Most of us will never approach a four-minute mile or two-and-a-half hour marathon, but I truly believe that if done correctly, *anyone* can learn to love running. And perhaps more inspiring, just about anyone (that's you!) can train themselves to run a 5K, a half marathon, a marathon, or even an ultramarathon (any race longer than 26.2 miles). You read that right—just about anyone.

You, the Marathoner?

There's a secret about distance running that people who think they hate it don't understand. Ready?

Running a 5K (3.1 miles) isn't three times harder than that gym-class mile was, and running a marathon isn't even close to 26.2 times as hard as that mile.

Why? Because nobody could possibly keep up their gym-class mile intensity (and misery) for much longer than that one mile. That was an all-out effort, and it was often the *only* running we did all year! If you're not in shape and haven't built up your aerobic system and your endurance, then of course running hard for eight or ten minutes is going to feel terrible.

But to run a marathon, a half marathon, or even a 5K—and more importantly, to endure the months of training that go into it—everything about your running must change, from your mindset to your form. And that makes endurance running an entirely different (and much more comfortable) experience than that gym-class mile ever was.

I once heard Brendan Brazier, the vegan professional Ironman triathlete, say that the longer an endurance event is, the more the race becomes about the quality of your training and the less about your natural talent. That's how Brendan was able to become a pro athlete—as a kid, he understood that if he worked hard enough and was smart about his training and diet, he could become a pro Ironman triathlete (an Ironman requires its participants to swim 2.4 miles, bike 112 miles, and if that weren't enough, run a marathon to cap off the day).

This is a remarkable distinction, with an incredibly inspiring implication! It means that as average Joes and Janes, we're far more likely to perform well—and enjoy the profound benefits to our lives that come from proving to ourselves just how much we're capable of—if we focus on the very events that appear the most daunting. I'm talking about endurance events, like half marathons, marathons, and beyond—awe-inspiring distances to the average person on the street who likely won't run that far all year!

> *Demonstrating to yourself that your body is capable of running long past what you probably think is the breaking point can work absolute wonders for your confidence, your motivation, your body—in short, your entire life.*

This is why I love running and endurance training in general. And it's why I hope you'll give it a chance, even if somewhere along the line you've gotten the idea that you're not built for this sort of thing. Demonstrating to yourself that your body is capable of running long past what you probably think is the breaking point can work absolute wonders for your confidence, your motivation, your body—in short, your entire life.

And as another bonus: if your interest as a vegetarian or vegan is in spreading the message, what better way to inspire your family, friends, and coworkers than by doing something the "old you" would have thought impossible?

Like a Fine Wine . . .

There's one more reason running is a fantastic choice of sport for getting fit and staying that way for the rest of your life. It's that, in a way, running favors age. As runner and author Joan Ullyot put it, "No matter what your age when you start running, you can expect about 10 years of improvement. That's how long it takes to learn the game."

Hear that? *No matter what your age.* If you look at aggregate marathon statistics year-to-year, you'll see something remarkable: Runners aged forty-five to forty-nine consistently average faster finish times than those in the twenty-to-twenty-four age group. How can this be? Surely those twenty-somethings are fitter, more durable, and more energetic, right?

Perhaps. But in general, they don't have the experience that older runners do, and with endurance sports, experience trumps youth.

The reason is that running, like other endurance sports, is more cerebral than it lets on. As you run, you learn. And not just the obvious, conscious distinctions, like when and what to eat and drink and what pace is right for the distance you're running, but also subtle skills, like interpreting the messages your body is sending you—such as the heaviness in your legs 15 miles into a marathon that tells you to ease up if you plan on finishing this race. And there's an even deeper level of improvement, one that comes more from the mind than the muscles: With every stride you take, your brain improves at directing your legs to propel you forward, and over time, running becomes easier as you become more efficient (even without paying much attention to form).

> *With every stride you take, your brain improves at directing your legs to propel you forward, and over time, running becomes easier as you become more efficient.*

If you're searching for a sport that you'll be able to improve at for a long time to come (and one that's more physically demanding than riding around in a golf cart), look no further than running.

Let's get started. Here's how you can learn to love running and make sure running loves your body, too.

(As a side note, because running is my sport and exercise of choice, I'll use it as the example throughout the book. But if you prefer another sport, especially an endurance sport, such as cycling, swimming, or triathlon [the combination of all three], you should be able apply the advice here to help you get started.)

NOT JUST FOR ENDURANCE ATHLETES: How Plant-Based Eating Benefits Bodybuilders, Too

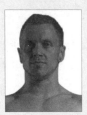

By Ed Bauer
Champion Vegan Bodybuilder and Owner of PlantFit Training Studio, plantfitpdx.com

I initially went vegan in 1996 at the age of sixteen when I learned of the cruelty involved when using animals for food. This commitment to living a compassionate lifestyle has kept me 100 percent vegan, but the health benefits have always seemed like an added bonus. As an athlete, I have realized that I may have a benefit over traditional omnivores because of my ability to recover faster.

In all the years of being vegan, my approach to nutrition has surely evolved. When I first started, I remember eating Fritos and animal crackers for lunch, not exactly a healthy meal. I now understand the importance of eating plant-based, nutrient-dense, whole foods for truly being at the top of my game. I wish I learned about healthier food sooner. For the first ten years of being vegan, I hardly, if ever, ate kale, avocado, quinoa, beets, tempeh, flax-seeds, or pumpkin seeds. Now, these are all some of my favorite foods. Seeds

NO MEAT
ATHLETE

specifically seemed to be the missing ingredient that helped me increase my strength across the board.

As a personal trainer, CrossFit athlete, and bodybuilder, the idea of veganism is still scoffed at in the fitness industry. This motivates me more to show the power of a plant-based diet. I do this through competing in bodybuilding and CrossFit competitions. I plan on running my first marathon this year as well! When people see what I can accomplish and what I look like, it speaks loud and clear to them that a plant-based diet does not hinder your health, looks, or performance in any way. I encourage you to adopt this lifestyle and see what you can accomplish. The sky is the limit!

Find Your Inspiring Obsession

Before you read any further, whether you're already a runner or not, I'd like you take out a piece of paper. We're going to have some fun. (Come on, do it! This is the most important part of the whole book!)

I want you to allow yourself to think big for a few minutes, to ignore whatever limitations you have in your head about what you're capable of, and to give yourself permission to dream.

That's right, we're going to set a goal. We're going to set one single goal that will become your driving force, the thing that right now is far out of reach and whose achievement will require you to change and improve.

Because we're in the running and fitness section of the book, that's where I'd like you to focus. You can always go back and set a dietary goal, too ("I'll become a weekday vegan within three months," "I'll eat raw for a month," etc.), but I think right now it's best to choose a single, primary goal, and eventually set related goals that will aid in achieving it.

Right now let's just focus on something athletic-related that you would absolutely love to achieve.

Note the wording there: *absolutely love to achieve.* I mean it!

Setting Your Goal Too Low Is Worse than Setting It Too High

For a lot of people who have never run before, I'd wager that the first thing that pops into their heads when I mention a goal is "run a 5K." If that's what you thought of, let's look at it closer: Does the idea of being able to run a 5K, and the level of fitness you'd need to possess to do it, give you butterflies in your stomach and make your palms sweat a little?

If so, fantastic. Those are good signs that a 5K might just be the right goal for you, right now. But I suspect that for many people for whom a 5K seems like a "reasonable" goal to start with, it isn't exciting enough to really get you jazzed up. If, when you think about setting the goal to run a 5K, you think, "Yeah, the training might be tough sometimes, but I could see myself doing that," then it's not exciting enough. Come on, think really big!

I always know that I've set a good goal when something about it scares me.

Would a 10K (6.2 miles) be more inspiring? What about a half marathon? What about a *full marathon*? A triathlon? What would be so motivating that when your head hit the pillow at night, you couldn't wait to wake up so you could keep making progress toward it? I'm not encouraging you to be foolhardy here—once you've thought of a goal, we'll examine it a little closer to make sure it's right for you. And absolutely, whatever goal you decide on, we're going to make sure to set a reasonable deadline to give yourself plenty of time to work up to your goal. But what we're not going to do is limit whatever that ultimate desire of yours is.

I always know that I've set a good goal when something about it scares me. It might be the goal itself: when I decided to run my first fifty-miler, I was literally afraid of doing it. I was scared of how much physical pain I would have to experience on race day to keep going after thirty or forty miles when I wanted to stop more than anything in the world—except for one thing, of course, which was to finish.

But other times, the fear isn't of the goal itself, but of what your friends or family might say when you tell them about your goal (which by the way, you'll need to do). It's nice to think that we surround ourselves with supportive people. But I know a goal is worthwhile when I'm actually kind of embarrassed to tell people about it—and not just because of the natural fear of failure and the humiliation failing would bring. More than that, the fear is that friends and family will laugh at you for even daring to think you could achieve what you've just told them about! When you feel that kind of afraid, you know you're onto something that could change everything for you.

This is what the Boston Marathon was for me. When my college buddies and I set out to run our first marathon and decided we wanted to qualify for Boston in the process, of course our other friends laughed. But it was in good fun, and I can't blame them: They had every reason to doubt us. We were brand-new to running, and here we were thinking we were going to achieve something that so many serious runners fail to ever do!

But after that first marathon, after we limped across the finish line with a time 103 minutes slower than what it would have taken to qualify for Boston, and after I truly understood just how daunting a task it is to even run a marathon (much less finish under three hours and ten minutes to qualify), that's when it became a real goal. After turning in the time that I did, it was almost embarrassing to go around telling people I planned to qualify for Boston. But the fact that I wasn't ashamed—because I had made myself so certain that I would do this one day—is what I now can see was the biggest edge I had going for me. (It certainly wasn't my ability as a marathoner!)

I want you to choose something like what Boston was for me. Something that you currently cannot do, something that will force you to grow inside and out.

It took me seven years to qualify for Boston, but your goal absolutely doesn't have to take you that long. My goal to run a fifty-mile ultramarathon, which I mentioned earlier, is another good example of something that felt huge and out of reach at the time I set it, and it took only six months or so to come to fruition.

HOW TO BE A NO MEAT (TRI) ATHLETE, ONE STEP AT A TIME

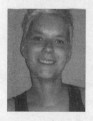

By Tina Žigon

I have been a vegetarian for almost twenty years and vegan for more than six of those. Although I am grateful for all the health and environmental benefits a plant-based diet provides, I eat the way I do mainly for ethical reasons.

I was never a sporty type. I used to be one of those "cool" kids who refused to run laps or participate in any other sport-related activities. I always liked watching sports, but I thought one had to be born with some sort of a talent to be able to actually participate.

All this completely changed during a 2010 Thanksgiving dinner when my girlfriends talked me into signing up for a sprint-distance triathlon with them.

(continued)

I still don't know how they managed to do that. To be honest, when the buzz from the wine I drank during dinner wore off, I was still excited, but mostly terrified. But because I am a stubborn person who finishes everything she commits to do, I was ready to take on the challenge.

I went to my first spin class, and then the second and third one, and then I stopped counting. On a snowy, cold day in January 2011, I went to an indoor track with my husband, a longtime runner, to run for the first time. At that point, I wasn't able to run one-third of a mile before having to stop and gasp for air. I could barely walk the next day, yet I was determined to keep on going.

I still remember my first runner's high—it was the most amazing experience I've ever had. And I also loved the progress I kept noticing. Being able to run a mile, then two, then three. In April that year, I ran my first 5K. Then a 5K trail run in May. I bought a bike. I started swimming. And in August 2011, I finished my very first sprint-distance triathlon!

Perhaps my description makes it all sound easy. It wasn't and it still isn't. But because I had made a commitment to do that triathlon, I couldn't give up. Especially because I also told the whole world that I had signed up for that race. I am also lucky to have such a supportive husband and an awesome, inspiring, and encouraging group of friends. When the going got tough, I turned to one or all of them for support and advice. I still do.

After that triathlon, I decided to run more. I signed up for the Buffalo half marathon. I trained for it using the *No Meat Athlete Half Marathon Roadmap*, and in May 2012, I finished it. It was the most difficult thing I've ever accomplished, but I'm already signed up to run another one. I also finished two more sprint triathlons and was thrilled to achieve a personal record in the last one. I'm eyeing an Olympic distance now, and I want to do a whole marathon someday. I am now that crazy person who doesn't mind getting up really early to run a five-mile turkey trot before starting the other Thanksgiving activities.

It is still hard to believe how much has changed for me in just two years. I can't even imagine my life without running now (biking and swimming, too, but especially running). And though it's been two years since I took those first steps on a running track, and I've run many miles since then, I am still in awe every time I go for a run. I'm in awe of how amazing our bodies are and what kind of challenges they can endure and overcome if we only give them a chance. I'm in awe of myself and my humble beginnings and how far I've gotten by just putting one foot in front of the other, no matter how difficult it is to do that sometimes. My life is definitely better now than it was two years ago, and I am proud to call myself a no meat (tri)athlete.

A Warning about Attainable Goals

A lot of people have had the unfortunate experience of being taught about S.M.A.R.T. goals (specific, measurable, attainable, relevant, time-bound).

I'm sure some of S.M.A.R.T. is actually, well, smart, but let me tell you something: "Set attainable goals" is the most limiting advice I've ever heard when it's interpreted the way most people interpret it. The real point of this maxim is to prevent you from becoming overwhelmed—for some people, setting too big a goal discourages them because they know deep down that they'll never get there. But most people don't need to worry about setting too big a goal; what we need to watch out for is the tendency to play it safe. Most people never take any action because they set their goals too low— they set goals that don't excite them to the core.

I suppose one could argue that qualifying for the Boston Marathon (for me) was attainable, while, say, trying to win an Olympic gold medal would not have been. Fair enough, but where do you draw the line? For me, Boston sure didn't feel achievable at the time I set out to do it! Back then, most people probably would have argued that taking, say, fifty-three minutes off my marathon time to get down to four hours was an attainable goal, but running a 3:10 marathon (*another* fifty minutes faster!) was not. I had no reason to think I could ever train myself to hold a 7:15 mile-per-minute pace for 26.2 miles when, at the time, I couldn't hold that pace for even one mile! It's a good thing I was "unreasonable" and didn't listen to anyone who told me what I was trying to do was impossible.

I'd rather you set a goal that's too lofty and make a ton of changes but ultimately fall short, than aim too low and never get motivated enough to start.

If you set a goal that feels very attainable, not much changes because it's something you know you can achieve, thus there's no need to take any massive action, no need to crash through your perceived limits or transform yourself into the incredible person you'd have to be to achieve that goal.

> *Most people never take any action because they set their goals too low— they set goals that don't excite them to the core.*

When you set a goal that seems impossible, though, that's when the magic happens. First, you get insanely excited because it's something you've never dared to lust after before, out of fear of failing. It energizes you just to think, "What if, just maybe, somehow . . . ?"

Then you recognize that, yes, it is impossible—right now. There's a tremendous gap between where you are and where you want to be, and to close that gap, your whole life will have to change. And *that*—how you'll need to change and the person you'll need to become to achieve your goal—is the real point of setting your sights on something incredible.

If you're hung up on attainable versus unattainable, just forget about it and instead apply this simple test: Does your goal inspire you? Does it make you want to get out the door right now to get to work? If not, find the level of goal that will inspire you the most. If it's too lofty, you'll know because you won't be motivated to do anything. Likewise if it's too small. When it's right, you'll know because it motivates you into action.

I'll add one disclaimer here, an exception to what I've just stated. The one time I do like the requirement of "attainability" is when it comes to the time frame in which you'd like to reach your goal. It's said that most of us overestimate what we can achieve in a year, but drastically underestimate what we can achieve in a decade, so don't fall into the trap of hoping for dramatic changes before you've had the chance to put in the work.

Shoot for the stars, sure, but give yourself a reasonable amount of time to reach them.

I've often failed at reaching my goals because I didn't set the time frame far enough in the future. Often, the temptation to set a really short time frame for doing something far beyond your present ability is a result of laziness (simply not being willing to work for a long time at achieving your goal) or even a form of self-sabotage. For example, if you told yourself you wanted to make it to the Olympics in ten years, you'd be in for ten years of immensely hard work. But tell yourself you're going to do it in six months and deep down, you know that effort will burn you out and give you an excuse to quit.

Sometimes, when I've experienced failure as the result of aiming to achieve a goal too quickly (such as when I failed at qualifying for the Boston Marathon the first six times), I've avoided getting discouraged and simply set the goal again, with more motivation than ever. But more often, the initial failure took the wind out of my sails and I've abandoned goals that at one time meant a lot to me. Shoot for the stars, sure, but give yourself a reasonable amount of time to reach them.

Stop Setting Goals and Start Making Decisions!

I've used the word "goal" up until now because it's familiar. But setting goals is not really what you should be doing—instead, you should be *making decisions*.

I know it sounds like a stupid language device that won't really make any difference five minutes from now, but I promise it's more than that.

When you set a goal, that goal is something you're hoping for. It's the target, and you're going to shoot for it. But when you make a real decision, your whole persona shifts. Once you decide that you're going to do something (no matter what happens!), in some way it's as if you've already done it. You start acting and thinking like a person who could achieve it, and that's a heck of a lot different than just hoping.

Let's Set a Huge Fitness Goal, Right Now

Here we go. Let's get started now. And again, please make sure you actually do this! Don't just read passively; reading alone will never get you anywhere. It's action that makes the difference.

STEP 1: GET SOME DREAMS ON PAPER.

Right now, give yourself permission to be like a kid writing a Christmas list. Take five minutes to write down every accomplishment that excites you, focusing (for now) on physical health and fitness. Remember, don't limit yourself. We'll look closer at these in the next steps, but for now, put down everything you can imagine wanting to do, no matter how long it'll take. Keep writing for the whole five minutes, don't let your pen stop moving!

One caveat: I'd encourage you not to set weight-loss (or weight-gain) goals. Though those results are often happy consequences of other goals, no number is going to inspire you enough to get out the door to train, time and time again, even when it's raining out and you had a rough day at work and all you want to do is lie on the couch and watch TV.

Would running a half marathon for a charity that's deeply meaningful to you get you excited? How about running a 10K with your spouse? A marathon relay with three runner friends? Competing in a Tough Mudder or other obstacle race? Beating your favorite celebrity's marathon time? Running the 135-mile Badwater Ultramarathon? Running half an hour without stopping? How about running a destination marathon in another country?

And remember, although I'll focus mainly on running in this book, there's no reason you should limit yourself to running. What about finishing an Ironman triathlon? Completing a century (100 miles) bike race? A fifty-mile bike race?

This is about what inspires *you*! Go wild with it.

STEP 2: CREATE A TIMELINE FOR EACH GOAL.

Go through your list and next to each item, estimate how long it'll take you to achieve each goal. Be optimistic, but be realistic. You don't need to be too specific yet, just write down "six months," "one year," "five years," "fifteen years," etc.

STEP 3: CIRCLE YOUR TOP THREE ONE-YEAR GOALS.

Choose the three goals that, if you could accomplish them all within a year, would transform you as a person, whether that transformation shows up in your body or your character.

Don't choose more than three because it's too easy to get overwhelmed. And now put a star next to the one that's your main, "banner" goal—the one that, even if it was the only goal you accomplished this year, would still be pretty darn incredible. For example, if your main goal is a half marathon, perhaps your other two will be stepping stones along the way, like first running for a half hour without stopping and later running a 10K.

STEP 4: GET SPECIFIC ABOUT YOUR THREE ONE-YEAR FITNESS GOALS.

Specificity is crucial. We don't want to be vague here. "Run more" would be a pretty useless goal (and this is why so many New Year's resolutions are forgotten in the first week of January).

Make sure each of your goals has a deadline, whether it's a full year in the future or something you plan on doing within three or six months. And if adding details makes your goals more exciting or easier to visualize (say, a specific race or location or who will be there to share it with you), by all means add them. Just don't let these additional specifications become so detailed that your goal is no longer within your control (like requiring that it's sunny and cool on your race day).

Another crucial component is your "why." Having a strong enough reason to achieve a goal, at first, is so much more important than the "how." Very often, the "how" takes care of itself once you believe that what you set out to do simply must happen. Under each goal and the details about it, write down a few sentences about why you're absolutely committed to seeing it through to its achievement—why you simply *must* do it.

You'll want to review and think about these goals as often as possible, ideally every day, and remind yourself of the "why" at least once a week. I like to do little things, like setting an image from my goal race's website as the background on my computer or even cutting out an ad for the race from a magazine and putting it in a place where I'll see it every day. It's not that I want to sit and visualize myself running the race without taking any action. Instead, I want to have a reminder, in a place where I won't miss it, that serves to motivate me and help me stay focused on my outcome.

Get specific about what it is you're going to do and then write it down, find photos on the Web, or do whatever will motivate you most and remind you daily about your commitment.

STEP 5: MAKE PLANS AND TAKE AN ACTION.

If you were to stop at Step 4, you'd be far more likely to achieve these goals than if you had simply let them remain thoughts in your head. By putting pen to paper, you've taken a big step toward transforming these desires from thoughts into outcomes. But you can go far beyond this, right now, by making plans and starting with the first real-world action toward the achievement of each goal.

Again, let's take the example of a half marathon, assuming you can run a mile or so right now but not much farther. The first thing I'd do in this situation is find a race that will work with your time frame. Once you've got it, pull up a calendar and figure out how many weeks you've got until the race. Then look at some training plans and figure out how long they are (many are twelve weeks) and how far you need to be able to run before you start the plan (many require that you've been running twelve to fifteen miles a week for a month or two before you start). Then think about how your other goals fit into this plan. Perhaps you can time your first 10K to happen four months before your half marathon, for example.

Continue working backward in this way all the way to the present moment, where you can use the principles of habit change described earlier and in the next chapter to get started.

Finally, take one action (today!) to start making your main goal real. If you're brave, put your money on the line and sign up for your race. Or tell someone about your goal and enlist them to help keep you focused.

Congratulations! You've drawn a line in the sand and declared that you're going to make this happen! Can you feel how much closer this fitness goal—and the person you'll need to develop into—is to becoming a reality, now that you've made a real decision about it?

Great. Give yourself a pat on the back for making this decision and taking the first step, and when you're ready, we'll discuss in the next chapter how to make running a habit so that you don't need to rely on willpower alone to keep you motivated.

CHAPTER 7

HOW TO MAKE RUNNING A HABIT

Just like we did with healthy eating, we're going to approach running as a habit to be formed, and we'll use what we know about the process of creating habits to maximize your chances of success. This will mean the following:

1. Choosing a daily trigger

2. Starting small

3. Making it enjoyable

4. Recording and rewarding

5. Not trying to change other habits at the same time

Later in the chapter we'll get into more technical matters, like running form and types of workouts, but first, let's see how to apply each of these guidelines to running.

1. Choose a Daily Trigger

You don't have to run or exercise every day. Once you get into the habit and start serious training, you'll find a day off (or even several) each week will give your mind and body a chance to rest and recover.

But when you're starting out, making your exercise a daily routine will lessen the time it takes for it to become automatic. To aid in that process, we want to identify a daily trigger or cue that will tell your brain it's time to exercise.

Your trigger should be something that happens once every day, without fail. It could be waking up in the morning, brushing your teeth, taking your lunch break, or getting home from work. As long as it happens every day, automatically, then it'll work.

Once you find your trigger, you want to get outside for your run (or walk) immediately after it happens. This will begin to teach your brain, "Once X happens, do Y," with Y in this case being running or walking.

Don't skip this step! The trigger or cue is an essential part of the habit cycle, and without a well-defined trigger, your habit will never be quite as ingrained as it could be.

2. Start Small

Small means really small. If you're out of shape or you've never done much running, this probably means doing some walking at first. Which is fine—swallow your pride and understand that every time you lace up your shoes and get out the door, you're building the neural pathway that will eventually become an automatic habit of exercising.

You'll need to decide for yourself how much is enough, but I urge you to err on the side of making it too easy and too short. Remember, right now we're not trying to make significant physical changes—instead, we just want to do what it takes to build the habit at first, without draining your willpower by making it too demanding.

If you're starting from scratch, five minutes of walking is plenty. If you find that amount is causing you to procrastinate, you can do even less! Try two minutes or even just putting on your shoes and going outside.

Stick with this initial amount for a week before you think about increasing it, and only if you've been able to do your exercise every day for a week should you allow yourself to increase the amount or intensity.

There's another reason to start small: in addition to what it'll do for your chances of making your running habit stick, it's the best way to avoid injury! Your legs need time to adapt to the stresses that even easy running puts on them, and forcing yourself to do less than you might feel up to in the early stages is an insurance policy against overuse injuries that can result from too quickly increasing your mileage.

Every time you lace up your shoes and get out the door, you're building the neural pathway that will eventually become an automatic habit of exercising.

If you're already in decent shape, you can do more than five or ten minutes, but don't overdo it. When I'm coming back from a long time without running (and yes, I go through these slumps like anyone else), twenty minutes of easy running each day for a week is how I start. Then each week I add five or ten minutes to the daily run until I'm back to a mileage level I'm comfortable with.

HIGH-ENERGY MEALS TO POWER YOUR WORKOUTS

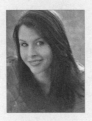

By Erika Mitchener
Personal trainer and Nutrition Coach, Worcester, Massachusetts
www.epowerliving.com

One thing I learned how to do when I transitioned to eating a plant-based diet is planning all my meals for the week and spending two days preparing them. I usually will prepare my meals on Sunday and again on Wednesday (I switch my menu up on Wednesdays). This took the guesswork out of trying to learn a new vegan meal every day or being stuck when I'm in a hurry and don't have time to cook.

When it comes to the gym and lifting weights, being vegan is confusing to some people. They think that vegans are weak or can't build muscle because we don't eat meat. If they want to learn, I take the time to explain where I get my nutrients. I often will write out a quick meal plan and recommend some of my favorite cookbooks, websites, and of course, the documentary *Forks Over Knives*. I've helped quite a few friends take a six-week vegan challenge or just taught them how to get enough protein from other sources besides animals.

My favorite workout meals include the following:

- Pre-workout: banana, dates, and some quinoa, with a few walnuts or almonds for fat and protein.

- Post-workout: sweet potato, sautéed kale and greens, and barbecued tempeh.

- My favorite smoothie recipe is my green full meal smoothie: A handful of baby spinach, 1 banana, 1 pear, 2 dates, lemon juice, 1/4 cup (20 g) oats, 1 tablespoon (12 g) flaxseeds, 1 scoop of Sun Warrior vanilla protein powder, 1 tablespoon (8 g) maca, and enough water to reach desired consistency.

3. Make It Enjoyable

Again, we're trying to eliminate the need for willpower right now. You want the experience of running to be as much fun (or at least as painless) as possible while you're forming the habit. And the easiest way to do that is to slow down.

Who said that every run has to be done as fast as possible? This idea is left over from gym class, and you'll do best by banishing it from your thoughts.

What most people mean when they say they "hate running" is that they hate running fast. So slow down—way down. Go ahead and find your Easy pace (capitalized because we'll refer to it often later), which is the speed at which you can pretty easily carry on a conversation, your mouth doesn't drop open, and you're relaxed. For now, don't worry about measuring your heart rate or actual speed for this Easy pace, just listen to your body and feel yourself in this zone.

If you've never run before or you're out of shape, then this Easy pace is likely a walk or perhaps a brisk walk that's not quite a run. Even for experienced runners, Easy pace often borders on shuffling, which makes you wonder what people who drive by must be thinking.

Easy pace isn't terribly exciting, but if all you've ever done is run hard, then your first run at this speed will be an eye-opener. You'll realize that, if you had to, you could keep this pace up for a pretty long time. I remember how light and free I felt when I first realized that if I just slowed down, I could run for three or four miles without stopping, when prior to that, one mile was about my limit before I'd start gasping for air.

Even experienced runners will benefit from the introduction of Easy-pace runs to their training, and if you're just getting restarted, they're a great way to ease back into it.

If you're used to running an eight-minute mile for your workouts, slow it down to nine or ten minutes per mile and just focus on enjoying how it feels to be moving without straining. If the farthest you've run at your old pace is a 5K, just imagine how far you could go at this slower one.

Running slow is an entirely different experience, both mentally and physiologically, than running fast. And as you practice it, you'll learn to feel your Easy pace without thinking about it, and you can let your mind wander. Enjoy the outdoors, listen to your breathing, or use this relaxed state to tap into the enhanced creativity it encourages and think through what's going on at home or work. (Just ask Einstein, who said of his theory of relativity, "I thought of it while I was riding my bicycle.") Who knew exercise could be so relaxing?

And running slowly isn't the only way to make the experience more enjoyable. Some people like listening to music while they run, and as long as you're able to hear other runners and traffic, there's nothing wrong with that. If you find that anything you're wearing is uncomfortable, do yourself a favor and replace it with a running-specific version from the running store. Running clothes aren't cheap, but if a little comfort makes the difference between sticking with this habit (and ultimately improving your health and fitness) or giving it up, then it's worth the price.

Finally, what if Easy-pace running isn't enjoyable for you? What if you're a type-A personality who thrives on speed and challenge and achievement? Well, you've still got to go easy on your body if you're just getting into running, but because the point is to make it fun, do what it takes to have fun. If that means working in thirty seconds of sprinting after every three minutes of Easy-pace running, do it.

4. Record and Reward

After the trigger and the activity itself, the step that completes the habit cycle is the reward. If you want to create a habit and get past the point of having to work up the willpower to run every time, then you've got to ensure that your brain feels a sense of pleasure when you're finished.

The simplest way to do this is to write down your accomplishment on a chart. Placing a single "X" in a box that signifies you completed your activity today can be deeply gratifying, especially if it's in a highly visible place where you'll see it throughout the day. If you want to get fancier, you can log your progress on a site like Daily Mile (www.dailymile.com) or just post it on Facebook for your friends to see that you did your exercise. Whichever way of recording you choose, do it as soon as possible after you complete your run so that your brain knows the two events are related.

The act of tracking your progress, by the way, independent of its role as a reward, can do wonders for you. Business people know that whatever outcomes are focused on and tracked will tend to improve, even without a conscious effort to do so. In his book *The 4-Hour Body,* author and entrepreneur Timothy Ferriss tells the story of a man who lost twenty-eight pounds simply by tracking his weight each day, even when he was very careful not to make any conscious changes to his diet or exercise habits! Apparently, the awareness of tracking his weight each day and recording it led to tiny, subconscious changes that over time helped him to lose weight.

But you can go beyond tracking as your reward to increase your sense of satisfaction and accomplishment. I once saw an interview with *The Power of Habit* author Charles Duhigg, in which he suggested that eating a little piece of chocolate after your initial

> *Placing a single "X" in a box that signifies you completed your activity today can be deeply gratifying, especially if it's in a highly visible place where you'll see it throughout the day.*

workouts could help you form the habit even if the extra calories more than make up for those burned during exercise. Although in the long term, a reward like this would be counterproductive, the point is that in the beginning, it's not the physical benefits we're concerned about, but instead, the formation of the habit.

In the best case, you'll do Step 3 (Make it Enjoyable) well enough that the activity itself is the reward, and even if it's not this way at first, you might be surprised at how quickly you start to look forward to your run each day.

HOW I WENT PLANT-BASED, BEAT CHRONIC STOMACH PAIN, AND FINISHED MY FIRST ULTRA-MARATHON AND IRONMAN 70.3

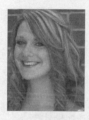

By Tori Brook

For more than five years, I had suffered from chronic stomach pain. I had seen two primary care physicians and multiple GI specialists, had food allergy testing, and gone through more "oscopies" than I care to remember, and yet nothing of concern was ever found. I was prescribed a long list of medications for everything from stress to digestive issues and still, nothing helped.

I tried my best to just live with it, but I felt abnormal, uncomfortable, and frustrated.

I reached my breaking point a few years ago. At the time, I'd run a few half marathons and a marathon, but my training had always suffered because I often didn't feel well enough to do it. I'd been so focused on what was wrong with my health for so long, and I wanted to shift that focus to something productive. I decided to set three goals for myself: to get better, to run an ultramarathon, and to finish an Ironman 70.3. Obviously, the second two goals relied heavily on accomplishing the first one. Determined to find a solution, I decided to make changes to my diet and try to solve once and for all the problems I was having.

I eliminated dairy about five years ago at the onset of stomach pain. One of the first specialists I saw said that my symptoms sounded a lot like lactose intolerance. Although it helped, dairy definitely wasn't the main cause.

Then, over the next few years, I slowly phased out red meat, then chicken, and then turkey. I still ate eggs frequently. I was an endurance athlete, and I was sure that I needed the protein to power my workouts.

With every minor change, I saw a gradual improvement, and my stomach problems became less of a focus in my day-to-day life. I was working toward my goal to run an ultramarathon, and I was seeing dramatic improvements in my running.

Then, in August 2011, I experienced one of the worst episodes I've ever had. I had gone out to breakfast with the family and ordered an omelet. I came home and assumed the fetal position on the floor of my house. I felt absolutely awful. That's the day I decided to try a full vegan plant-based diet.

I bought a couple of books on eating vegan and read everything I could find about balancing a plant-based diet with an active lifestyle. I started reading *No Meat Athlete* for reassurance that I could properly fuel my body while continuing my journey with endurance sports. I made a commitment to myself to cook more and try new foods. I found joy in preparing meals and realized, despite years of believing it, I actually don't suck at cooking.

A lot of people ask me if I get bored with the foods I eat. Certainly not! I've found my meals are more colorful and flavorful than ever before. Without the fear of feeling physically ill, I've started to enjoy food again.

One of my biggest concerns was the effect a plant-based diet would have on my training. I was concerned that I wouldn't have the energy to put the miles into training that I wanted. That couldn't be further from the truth. Since transitioning to a vegan diet, I have set a personal record in every distance and found that I have more energy than ever before. I also achieved my goals and ran my first 50K and my first Ironman 70.3 in 2012, each without a moment of GI trouble.

The best part, by far, has been the way I feel. After years and years of seeing doctors and using drugs without any relief, I decided to take control of my health with a natural approach, and it worked. I still have bad days, but rarely ever. Going to a plant-based diet is hands-down one of the best decisions I've ever made.

5. Don't Try to Change Other Habits at the Same Time

One of the wonderful things about healthy habits is the way they stack on top of each other. Once you start getting in shape by exercising, often you start eating better simply because you don't want to screw up everything you've worked toward.

But be careful. It's easy to fall into the trap of trying to overhaul your entire life all at once: "Starting tomorrow, I'm going to exercise every day, stick to a strict diet, stop drinking coffee, and read for thirty minutes each night." Sound familiar? As exciting as it sounds and as motivated as you may be, attempting to change so much at once almost never works. It takes too much willpower, and after a few days (if you make it that long), that willpower is depleted, and all of your well-intentioned changes fall apart.

Instead, practice patience. Promise yourself that you'll focus on just this one new habit until it feels routine, which means at least two or three weeks, probably even more. If exercising this restraint is tough for you (it is for me!), one trick you can try that I've found helpful is to make a list of all the habits you're tempted to change right now and put them below "Running" on a tracking sheet. Simply having them written out in front of you, knowing that you'll take care of each when you get to it, alleviates some of the feeling of urgency to change right now. You can also use this list to get excited for the start date of the next habit you're going to change, and that makes it all the more likely you'll stick with it, as opposed to simply deciding that you're going to change something in the spur of a moment.

To summarize this final key: Focus on one change at a time. Be satisfied with running (or whatever your sport of choice is) right now and don't try to change everything else in your life until this one is automatic. There's no rush—keep in mind that if you could change just one habit a month, in three years you'd have thirty-six new habits and be transformed from the inside out.

The above steps are really all it takes to get started: trigger, small action (run or walk), reward—day in, day out. Make the action so small, so easy, and so enjoyable that you can't possibly skip it. If you find that you're procrastinating even a little bit, you've started with too much. Make it easier or shorter. Remember, the point right now is to reinforce that habit loop in your brain, and only once that's established should you worry about (gradually) increasing the intensity or volume of your training.

FROM NEVER WALKING AGAIN TO RUNNING MARATHONS

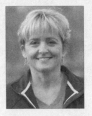

By Janet Oberholtzer

In 2004, I was almost killed when my body was crushed in a six-vehicle accident and the other five vehicles were semi-trucks. It took nine paramedics thirty-five minutes to cut me free from the debris. As they put me in the helicopter, my vitals were so low they assumed I wouldn't arrive at the hospital alive.

Doctors worked heroically to save my life and my almost-severed leg. I woke up twelve days later to discover that I might never walk again. My right leg had rods, screws, and pins in the shattered femur and ankle, my pelvis was fractured in so many places that the doctors dubbed it "Humpty Dumpty," and there was no guarantee how any of it would heal, especially my almost-amputated left leg.

Fast-forward eight years: I completed two full marathons within six months of one another on my own two feet. What happened? There was no overnight success, no spontaneous miracle, no quick recovery. It was a step-by-step, day-by-day, choice-by-choice recovery.

At first, I didn't grasp the extent of my injuries, but with time my pain, limitations, and deformed leg forced me to accept the reality of my new normal. Somewhere between the ongoing surgeries, therapy, and meds, I was sucked into the dark vortex of depression.

Finding myself debating whether life was worth living scared me enough to seek help from counselors. With their help, along with plenty of reading, I realized the power I have over my own life and I began doing what I could to enjoy life again.

I couldn't change what happened, but I had a choice in how I responded.

My hospital dietitian had said, "How you eat will determine how you heal." After researching what foods provide the most benefits, I switched to a plant-based diet. I soon noticed an increase in my energy, which helped me get off the couch to begin taking short walks and go on easy hikes.

With time, I was able to create a cycle of health: my diet gave me energy to exercise and the exercise made me crave healthy food and decreased my pain, allowing me to exercise more, which led to more healthy food, less pain, and more exercise.

That cycle of health is what took me from waking up in a hospital bed not knowing if I'd ever walk again to successfully doing two marathons. After the walks and hikes came biking and eventually running. Through trial and error, I found walking breaks are best for my beat-up body, so for any distance longer than ten miles I run three minutes, walk one minute, and repeat.

By doing what I can with what I have, where I am, I recovered better than anticipated and learned a few important things:

- Good food and exercise are essential for recovery and to maintain health.
- We are all capable of more than we give ourselves credit for.
- We have choices in how we respond to circumstances in our life.
- Some obstacles can be overcome and some we have to make adjustments for.

Life is too short to be miserable, so whether you've been run over by a truck or it only feels like you have, do what you can with what you have where you are!

The Basics of Good Running Form

To many people, the idea that we don't already know how to run is absurd. After all, we've done it since we were kids, so we should know how to run properly, right?

Well, it's true that if we could all run like we did when we were kids, we'd probably have beautiful, natural form. But the fact is that most people don't run that way anymore. Years of sitting at a desk for eight hours a day, injuries sustained from running or other sports, and going months or years with little to no physical activity have all changed our body mechanics for the worse. Add to these factors the heavy, cushioned shoes we've been walking or running around in, which allow us to change our stride to one that's totally unlike the way we naturally ran as kids, and running form becomes something that's worth at least a little time and attention.

But it doesn't have to be complicated. You can go as in-depth as you like, exploring entire programs designed to teach the most efficient form of running, but most philosophies about running form are pretty simple at their core and share several common elements. I've found that if you just focus on the primary keys that are taught in some form or another by all of these methods, you can develop a philosophy of running that is both simple and extremely effective—and for a beginner, I think that's more important than the nitty-gritty details of running form, about which there's no real consensus anyway.

As it turns out, there's an even simpler way to get at the heart of most modern approaches to running form—an approach to running that's decidedly old-school. And I mean prehistorically old.

What Barefoot Running Can Teach Us about Running Form

If you've paid any attention at all to the running world over the past few years, you've probably heard about the barefoot running craze or at least seen a few people walking around in Vibram FiveFingers, those funny-looking shoes with the toes. It's quite possible that the idea of running barefoot (or close to it) so that you can feel the ground and run the way nature intended is what brought you to running in the first place.

Although I wouldn't call myself a proponent of running exclusively barefoot or even in FiveFingers, I'm a big fan of the rationale that has made it so popular. Here's how the thinking goes.

Human beings have been running (primarily for the purpose of persistence hunting) for hundreds of thousands of years. And for the vast majority of that time, we've done it without shoes; the human foot has evolved over time into an incredibly advanced and efficient tool for the purpose.

When we run barefoot, then, we naturally assume the running mechanics that nature intended. We take quick, short strides, keeping our weight over our feet and landing on the midfoot or perhaps the forefoot. By running the way we were built to run, we're able to avoid injury, even over long distances.

When, instead, we run in fancy, high-tech, super-cushioned running shoes, we're all of a sudden able to run with an unnaturally long stride that forces us to come crashing down on our heels with each step. (Try landing hard on your heel without any protection, and you'll understand. On second thought, don't do that. It hurts.) Indeed, laboratory studies have shown that the impact shockwave through the leg is significantly higher in shod runners than in barefoot runners, despite the extra cushioning.

That's the theory, anyway. In practice, there are some other considerations that favor wearing at least some sort of protection on your feet. The most compelling, to me, is that we do so much of our running on rough roads now as opposed to the grass or dirt that the hunters who have inspired this way of thinking and running did.

The best advice I've heard for applying the principles of barefoot running in the modern world is this: *Run like a barefooter, but do it in shoes.* This means taking quick, light steps with your feet under your body instead of way out in front of you and landing on your midfoot instead of your heel. But more than just physically, the goal is also to run mentally like a barefooter: with the sense of playfulness and excitement that you see in kids when they run just because it feels good.

The best way to learn to run like a barefooter is to actually run barefoot for a few minutes—just some light barefoot jogging in the grass after your normal run can help you learn what it feels like. Have fun with it, but be careful because it's easy to twist your ankle if you're not used to running in the grass.

Once you've got the feeling, put your shoes back on, but try to recapture that feeling you had without shoes. It's not an easy thing to do, and if running barefoot appeals to you, by all means keep at it. The more you do it, the more the form will begin to carry over to when you're running in shoes.

But even if you have no desire to run barefoot regularly, we still want to work toward the form that barefooting imposes. Here, boiled down into three crucial but simple keys, is how to do that.

The Three Most Important Keys to Good Running Form

1. TAKE 180 STEPS EACH MINUTE.

The biggest change you can make to drastically lower the stress that running puts on your body is to take frequent steps. Like running slower, this isn't just a form of training wheels; it's a habit practiced by the best marathoners and ultrarunners in the world.

If you look at the leg turnover rate of most elite runners—that is, the rate at which they take strides—you'll find that nearly all of them take at least 180 steps per minute (three per second). Compare that to your average weekend warrior's stride rate, and you'll find that the elites are taking about twenty more steps each minute than the amateurs.

Why take more strides each minute? Because taking short, quick steps, as opposed to long, slow ones, means your feet spend less time in contact with the ground and create a smaller impact each time they do make contact.

How do you train yourself to take quicker steps? It's easiest to think of 180 steps per minute as three per second and then lock in with that rhythm as you stare at a ticking clock. Of course, this is far safer and easier on a treadmill than it is on the road.

Another way is to run to a metronome, or better yet, find a song with a tempo you can align your steps with. (See "Training Yourself to Take 180 Steps Per Minute" on the next page.)

It'll feel like the most awkward thing in the world at first, I promise. You'll feel like a cartoon character, spinning your wheels without actually covering much ground. But give it time. You're working different muscles than in any running you've done before, so it'll take some getting used to. But after several runs like this, it'll start to feel normal, and you'll be far less likely to get injured.

TRAINING YOURSELF TO TAKE 180 STEPS PER MINUTE

If you naturally run at far fewer than 180 steps per minute (three per second), running this way is going to feel really strange at first.

That's okay. These quicker, shorter strides will force you to use a whole new set of muscles, so it's to be expected that you'll feel *less* efficient until your body and muscles adjust. But trust me, it'll be worth it when you're running injury-free and tackling distances you've never before thought possible.

Let's first get clear on exactly what I mean when I say "180 steps per minute." I'm talking about the total number of impacts you make with the ground in one minute—that is, counting both feet. (Some people call this your cadence and measure the number of times a single foot hits the ground, so you might hear some people refer to this as a "cadence of ninety." It's the same thing.)

The easiest way to learn what this feels like is to think of it as three steps each second. Here's what I recommend you do:

- Get on a treadmill.
- Set it to a brisk but comfortable speed, a pace where you could speak a few sentences without difficulty but would have trouble carrying on a whole conversation (running really slowly for this is actually harder than running fast, at first).
- Start running and time your steps so that each time a second ticks, your third step impacts the ground.

For example, if your right foot lands when the clock shows one second (0:01), then it'll be "left," then "right" again before your left foot lands exactly when the clock hits 0:02. Then it"ll be "right," then "left" before your right foot hits on 0:03. And so on.

Once you get the hang of it, you'll find it's pretty easy to get into a rhythm—it's sort of like a waltz.

Now Get Comfortable with It

It takes a while for this pace to feel normal, but once you've done it for a while, it will. Assuming you won't always be running on a treadmill or staring down at your watch while you run, it's helpful (if you wear headphones while you run) to find a song whose beat matches this tempo, so that you can just run with the music.

The song I always recommend for this is Eric Johnson's "Cliffs of Dover", which is entirely instrumental but actually a pretty good song to run to (note that it doesn't get going until about forty-five seconds in). But you can find any other song that's roughly this tempo or even one that's half as fast—in that case, you just have to take two steps for every beat instead of one.

Finally, realize that you won't always need a crutch like a clock or headphones to achieve this rhythm. Eventually this turnover rate will be grooved, and it'll just be what you do naturally. I still glance down at my watch for two or three seconds every now and then to line my steps up, but if that's not your thing, imagine that you're running barefoot over broken glass to get the image of quick, light steps.

One More Thing: What about Speed?

More than just about anything else, this single tip compels people to email me and tell me how much it has helped them stop getting injured and run longer. But a question often comes up: How should this stride rate change when you want to run faster or slower?

The simple answer is it shouldn't. Keep this constant turnover rate of 180 steps per minute and adjust your running speed by changing your stride length. For slow, relaxed runs, you'll be taking very short steps, and when you want to open it up for a 5K or something even shorter and faster, you'll lengthen your stride so that you cover more ground with each step. But you're still taking 180 or more steps each minute at all speeds.

(Note: there's nothing magical about the exact number 180. If you can be somewhere in the neighborhood, or even considerably faster, you'll be fine.)

2. LAND ON YOUR MIDFOOT INSTEAD OF YOUR HEEL.

I've already explained how modern running shoes encourage us to land with what's called a heel strike. Without shoes, it's painful to land on your heel when you run. But throw on a pair of heavy, cushioned, expensive running shoes, and you're invincible! You can land on your heel all day long and not feel a bit of pain.

But there's something dangerous about this type of landing. If we're not really built to run with a heel strike, then cushioning the heel to avoid pain will only lead to more problems, often further up the leg in the knee or hip. When we're barefoot, the pain of a heel strike prevents us from taking such long strides where the only possibility is to land on the heel. But once the pain is eliminated by shoes, we're free to take that long stride, and suddenly we're running with a form that's nothing like what we're built for. Rather than keeping our weight over our feet, we begin to land with our foot out in front of the body— a position that leads to all sorts of problems over time.

Most of us aren't going to be running barefoot, so it's important to pay attention to how we land because we can't rely on pain to signal when we're running in a way that will ultimately lead to injury. (Although if you wear somewhat minimalist shoes, like the ones I recommend for most runners, you'll be able to feel more than you can with heavy, cushioned shoes.)

There's some debate, even among barefooters, over whether it's best to land on the mid-foot or the forefoot, assuming we all agree that severe heel striking is bad (not everyone in the running community agrees with this, by the way). I like a mid-foot strike for a few reasons: first, forefoot striking tends to lead to a lot of up and down movement of the body, which is wasted energy when the direction you really want to go is forward. Second, a midfoot strike is more natural for most runners, especially those used to years of heel striking, than landing on the forefoot.

This is a good time to bring up an important caveat: if you've been running a certain way all your life (or if you haven't been running at all), it's critical that you make any changes to your form *gradually*. When you change your form, you use different muscles than you're used to using, and these muscles need time to develop; otherwise, you'll risk serious injuries (stress fractures are common among people who suddenly start running barefoot without first building up their barefoot mileage slowly). It's also mentally tiring to focus on form for more than a few minutes at a time.

One way to slowly introduce improvements to your form is to spend just thirty seconds out of every five minutes on your Easy-pace runs practicing your new form for the first week. The next week, spend a minute out of every five and gradually increase in this manner until the new form comes naturally.

3. LEAN FORWARD FROM THE ANKLES, NOT THE HIPS.

Lots of runners lean forward, but too many do it from the wrong place: their hips. Leaning forward from the hips results in an inefficient, bent-over posture that invites injury. Instead, you want to keep a relatively straight line from your ankles to the top of your head and lean your entire body forward while maintaining that line.

You may have heard of the idea of falling forward when you run, letting gravity do the work. The forward lean accomplishes exactly this. It should feel like you're constantly falling forward, using each successive step to catch yourself, rather than the opposite feeling of driving from behind with your legs to keep yourself in motion. Make sure your shoulders stay slightly ahead of your feet while you're running—you'll bend from the ankles, not the waist, to achieve this.

GETTING STARTED WITH BAREFOOT RUNNING

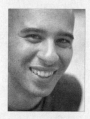

By Leo Babauta
Simplicity blogger at ZenHabits.net and vegan marathoner

For decades now, runners (including me) have been sold on the need for good running shoes—if you want to prevent injuries, invest in good shoes. You needed proper cushioning and sometimes rigid motion control or stability features, and if you had injuries, you probably had the wrong shoes.

But recent studies have proven what our ancestors have known all along: that running barefoot strengthens your feet and is a more natural way to run. Running in cushioned, motion-controlled shoes is like having your neck in a cast for a month—when you take the cast off, your neck muscles will be weak. You also pound your feet much harder with running shoes, causing problems not only with your feet, but also your knees and other joints. We're making our feet weak—it's no wonder we have all kinds of injuries. (There are numerous studies still being done on barefoot running versus running with shoes, so don't draw any long-term conclusions yet.)

Even more important than the strength of your feet is your connection to the earth. Simply put, shoes shelter us from the surfaces we run on, but that's not always a good thing. However, a big caveat: if you think barefoot running will make you faster, you're probably going to be disappointed. Running barefoot is about connecting with the ground, about feeling, about freedom and lightness, about fun. It's not about speed.

How to Get Started

In a word: slowly.

Many people make the mistake of doing too much, too quickly, which can lead to pain, injury, and discouragement. Remember, your feet, ankles, and calves are weak from running or walking in shoes all the time. You will find a lot of soreness if you go too far or too fast. You need to build it up slowly, gently.

—*(continued)*

Here's what I recommend:

1. Try running barefoot or with barefoot shoes like Vibram FiveFingers on a hard surface, just for a few minutes, slowly. Try this at the end of a regular run, if you're running consistently. Running on a hard surface is good for your first few times because you will naturally run with better form. With shoes, you're used to pounding on your heels and overextending your legs, but when you're barefoot, you have no cushion, and running by extending and pounding your feet on your heels is going to hurt on a hard surface. Run lightly, landing quietly and softly on your forefeet or midfeet. See more about form below.

2. Slowly lengthen the time you run barefoot (or with barefoot shoes). Increase just a minute or two longer, a few times a week. Go slowly and don't try to sprint or run hard. Continue to run lightly, working on not pounding. Try different surfaces, such as asphalt, concrete, grass, and dirt. Let your body adapt to this new running style and your muscles will slowly get stronger.

3. Eventually, you can do shorter runs completely in barefoot shoes. Shorter runs might mean fifteen to thirty minutes if you're an experienced runner or perhaps ten minutes for a less experienced runner. For longer or harder runs, you might still wear shoes because you're not ready for long or hard runs barefoot. Let this phase take several weeks.

4. Eventually you can stop using your running shoes. This is true especially if you have barefoot shoes and are used to running in them for longer runs. Your feet and legs should be stronger at this point. However, it might take a couple months to get to this point.

5. Gradually try running completely barefoot on softer or smoother surfaces. A park with a smooth concrete surface, or grass, or beaches are good places to start running without the barefoot shoes. Your soles are probably soft and sensitive if you've been using shoes most of your life, so it takes some adjustment to all of a sudden feel variable and rough surfaces under your feet. Starting out on rougher asphalt or surfaces with lots of pebbles (or worse, glass or pieces of metal) is a bad idea. I know—I tried it the first few times and it hurt! Eventually, you can do short to medium runs in bare feet.

Remember, at each stage, go slowly and take your time. There's no need to rush it, and even if you're feeling ambitious, hold back. It'll make the whole experience much, much more enjoyable.

The Barefoot Running Form

To run barefoot without pain, you'll probably need to adjust your form from the way you're accustomed to running with shoes (that's part of the point!):

- Land on your forefeet or midfeet (balls of your feet) instead of your heels. If you feel yourself landing on your heels, shorten your stride.

- Strides should be short. Don't extend your legs as far as you do with shoes. It should feel almost like you're running in place.

- Keep upright and balanced. Keep your feet under your hips and shoulders.

- Stay light. You should feel like you're light on your feet, not pounding at all. Barefoot runners tend to be a little more springy in their step than runners in shoes.

- Run quietly. If you are making a lot of noise with your steps (as shoe-wearing runners do), you're pounding too hard. Try to run softly, quietly, like an animal.

FOCUS ON THESE MENTAL IMAGES TO HELP YOU FIND YOUR FORM

If you focus on just the three principles we talked about previously, you'll be 95 percent of the way toward achieving an efficient running form. (In fact, you could get 80 percent of it just with the first key of taking 180 steps per minute.) But as you get more serious about running, you'll naturally start to wonder about other aspects of form. Rather than trying to remember a bunch of angles at which your joints should be bent, let's keep it simple, with a few easy-to-remember mental images. These aren't essential to get started, but if you're the curious type who isn't comfortable with just doing what comes naturally, you might find them helpful.

▶ Keep your hands lightly closed, as if you're holding butterflies and don't want to crush them.

▶ Envision that you have Tyrannosaurus Rex arms—not doing too much movement, just hanging out at your sides but bent with your hands in front of you.

▶ Pump your arms back and forth at your sides, not across your body.

WHAT ABOUT BREATHING?

For as integral to running (and almost all sports) as breathing is, the topic is oddly ignored among runners. Ask a runner, even a good one, how he or she breathes, and you'll likely get a shrug or maybe an answer of, "I don't really think about it; I just do what comes naturally."

> *For as integral to running as breathing is, the topic is oddly ignored among runners.*

Jack Daniels, a well-known running coach, recommends breathing with what's called a 2:2 rhythm: in for two steps, out for two steps (which means if you're running at 180 steps per minute, you're taking forty-five full breaths per minute). If there's a rule of thumb for how to breathe while you run, this is it.

But you may find that if you're training at a low intensity, you can actually breathe much more slowly than this without straining. In his fascinating book *Body, Mind, and Sport,* John Douillard suggests that by training yourself to breathe solely through your nose, you can decrease your breath rate to as little as fifteen breaths per minute. He argues that this is a much less stressful and more efficient way to run, especially at low intensities like what is required for a marathon or half marathon. Scott Jurek, the legendary vegan ultramarathoner, puts in another vote for nose-breathing in his book *Eat and Run*, and in fact mentions Douillard's book as one that he learned from.

If you decide to experiment with nose-breathing, understand that it takes time to get used to it. At first, you'll find it very hard to get enough oxygen without opening your mouth, especially on hills or when you pick up the pace. But with practice, nose-breathing can become second nature and so will a slower breath rate.

How to Begin Your Training

Now that we've covered the basics of a simple, efficient method of running, it's time to take it to the streets (or the trails, or the treadmill, or wherever you'll be doing your training). How you get started will depend greatly on your fitness and experience as a runner, but I'll provide a few guidelines here to help you decide what's best for your unique situation.

If You're Already a Runner

If you're already a runner and train regularly but you find yourself too often sidelined by injury or simply not progressing as well as you'd like, you can apply the running form suggestions here and the advanced techniques in the next chapter to your current training schedule. Keep in mind that changes in your form will take several weeks to feel comfortable, and you may even find that you become less efficient in the short term, as the burden of moving you forward shifts to new muscles that haven't had a chance to develop yet. But be patient; the rewards to running this way are great. Also, be sure to incorporate the form changes gradually—treat each of them as a new habit and use the habit change principles at the beginning of this chapter to incorporate them into your running so that they become automatic.

For example, if you use the technique from this chapter to calculate your current turnover rate and find that you're only taking 160 steps per minute, you might try doing one run each week on a treadmill so that you can get the sense of what it feels like to run at three steps per second as you align your steps with the clock on the treadmill for fifteen or twenty straight minutes. After two or three weeks, start incorporating this faster turnover into your normal runs, doing it for just one minute out of every five at first and then increasing that proportion each week until this faster cadence becomes second nature.

If you do nothing else I suggest in this chapter, I hope you'll try just two things: increase your turnover rate to 180 steps per minute and run your easy miles even easier than you already do. Those were the two keys that changed everything for me and allowed me to finally stop getting injured and put in the miles I needed to take serious time off my marathon, and I've seen them do the same for so many others.

If You're New to Running

If you're brand new to running or even if you've done some running in your life but it's been a while, I suggest you focus first on creating the habit of running. Go through the five habit change keys listed previously and create a plan for implementing the habit. You'll need to decide for yourself, for example, how much time or distance to start with and whether it's best to start out with walking. (For most people who have never run, I think it's best to swallow your pride and walk at first.)

An example of how someone who currently doesn't exercise, is slightly overweight, and has never run consistently might get started is as follows (this is just a general example, so adjust it any way you see fit).

1. Each day, as soon as you wake up or as soon as you get home from work, put on your running shoes and get out the door. (Start small, remember?)

2. Walk at a brisk pace for five minutes, perhaps with music if that makes the experience more enjoyable for you.

3. When you're done, make a big "X" on a calendar that's in a place where you'll see it often and do whatever else will make you feel great about it, whether that's posting about your run or walk on a social networking site or giving yourself a small reward.

4. If you do this for seven straight days (and only then!), allow yourself to do more. Increase the time to, say, eight or ten minutes.

5. If you succeed at this next level for seven straight days, allow yourself to do more. That might mean increasing to fifteen minutes or perhaps staying at ten minutes but jogging for three minutes in the middle.

6. In this way, gradually increase what you do each day, as long as you're having success and sticking with it. If you're missing days or procrastinating, stay at the current level or scale it back a bit and think about how you can engineer the experience so that it's more enjoyable or give yourself more accountability.

7. Once you can jog for about half an hour without stopping, congratulations! If you're not in 5K shape yet, you're very close, and you're ready to start incorporating different types of workouts into your training (and go for a 10K or half marathon, if that appeals to you).

Again, the right routine for you depends on you! The above example of starting with just five minutes of walking each day might be perfect for someone who hasn't exercised in years, but for someone who has hit the gym on and off for the past six months, chances are good that five minutes of walking is too little. For that person, perhaps running five minutes is the right place to start. It's up to you, and you'll know what works and what doesn't. Remember, it's fine to fail, and it's expected! Screw up, learn, and try again. Don't feel bad or guilty—just go back and figure out what didn't work last time, re-engineer your routine, and try again!

Because you're starting with a clean slate, you have the advantage of not having any bad habits to undo (well, at least when it comes to running form!). From the beginning, use the principles outlined in this chapter to ensure that you're using the form that will make running as comfortable and enjoyable as possible.

CHAPTER 8

TAKING IT TO THE NEXT LEVEL: ADVANCED TRAINING TECHNIQUES

So far, we've covered the basics of getting started with running, with most of our focus so far on form. Truthfully, there's not a whole lot more you need to know to train for a race and get yourself across the finish line. You could run the same, Easy pace for every workout, gradually building your endurance and the distance you could run without ever bothering to learn about the finer points of training.

But that's not quite what we're going for here. Sure, it'd be cool just to say you can run a distance that was unfathomable a few months prior, but being able to run far doesn't necessarily imply a high level of fitness. We want to focus on fitness, too, so we'll incorporate a variety of workouts into your training with the aim of burning fat, strengthening and building muscle, and improving cardiovascular health.

To close out the chapter, we'll cover the ins and outs of eating during and around your workouts. What you take in while you're running has an obvious effect on how you perform, but many new runners neglect the crucial few hours immediately before and after workouts, which are just as important for performance and recovery. Workout nutrition comes down to just a few simple guidelines about what to eat and when, so it's an easy way to take your training to a new level if you're not already paying attention to how you fuel your body.

The Basic Training Principle: Alternate Hard Workouts with Easy Ones

Easy pace will help you train to run far. But if you want to gain fitness or train to beat a certain time, then you've got to do some harder workouts so that your body can make adaptations and become stronger. (Besides, running at just one speed can get pretty boring.)

When you're ready to start mixing it up, you'll want to consider two other types of training to go along with the Easy pace: speed work and threshold training.

Before we get into the specifics of the different types of workouts, it's important to understand a critical principle that applies not just to running, but to all exercise. The way you build strength in a muscle is by working it hard and temporarily damaging the muscle fibers. The body responds by rebuilding the muscles and overcompensating by making them slightly stronger than before you tore them down. Assuming adequate nutrition, so that the body has the nutrients it needs to rebuild muscle tissue, this process takes anywhere from twenty-four to forty-eight hours. After several iterations of this process, the small gains begin to add up, creating noticeable improvement in strength, speed, and physical appearance (because you'll also burn fat as you exercise).

Here's the important consequence of the way this adaptation process works and the time it takes for your body to repair broken-down muscles: you must allow your muscles that time to rebuild before tearing them down again. If you work the same muscles too hard and too soon after a workout, before they've had a chance to recover, your workout will have been essentially wasted.

When it comes to running, the long and short of the above discussion is that you're not doing yourself any favors by working out hard (anything other than Easy pace) on consecutive days. This is the reason it's so critical that the Easy pace described in the previous chapter be, well, *really* easy—you want to get the aerobic benefit of logging in miles, but without interfering with the recovery of your muscles from the previous workout. Make your Easy runs too difficult, and you'll be sabotaging your own progress. And don't forget, because the heart is a muscle, too, even if you forego running entirely and choose to cross-train in between scheduled workouts, you've still got to take it easy on these days.

Along these same lines, I recommend taking one or two days completely off from running each week. Even when you're alternating Easy runs with more difficult ones, it's quite possible that certain muscles aren't fully recovering in between workouts, so giving them a day of complete rest every week will ensure that a recovery deficit isn't accumulating with each passing week.

Speed Work

Speed workouts are what they sound like. The goal is to run at a much faster pace than you could maintain for any significant distance, but to break up these bouts of intensity with rest intervals.

Speed work is generally done on a track, which has several benefits. First, the terrain is consistent and flat. Second, you can easily gauge your pace with a glance at your watch, and the markings on the track tell you how far you've run. But I know—heading to the track with a bunch of speedsters can be intimidating if you haven't set foot on one since high school. Luckily, there are less formal ways to do speed work if the track just isn't your thing, and we'll cover those here too.

THE BASICS OF THE TRACK

A standard outdoor track is 400 meters around, so it takes four laps to make a mile (technically, a mile is 1609.34 meters, but the difference is negligible for our purposes). This distance is measured along the inside lane, so you'll want to make that one your default lane, only moving to the other lanes to allow faster runners to pass (or if you're doing any racing where you're in an assigned lane).

Usually, runners coming up behind you on the inside lane will yell, "Track!" as they approach, signaling for you to move over if you haven't yet noticed them and done so on your own. You can do this, too, when you're the one passing, but keep in mind that not everyone knows what it means, so you may have to pass in the outside lanes from time to time.

Most of the time, you'll run counterclockwise around the track. Although shorter tracks inside gyms often alternate directions several times a week to help runners avoid injury from always turning the same direction, this isn't much of an issue with standard-length tracks. It's possible, especially if you run with a group where the coach or leader is always coming up with interesting workouts, that one day you'll find a reason to run clockwise around the track, but for the most part, just plan on running counterclockwise so as not to disrupt the flow of other runners.

There's a bold "Start" line on most tracks, and from there the track is marked with a line every 100 meters, dividing the track into four segments. Although none of the workouts from this book will have you running less than 400 meters at a time, the intermediate markings are helpful for gauging your pace. For example, if your goal is to run a 400-meter speed work interval in 100 seconds, then you'll want to use the markings on the track to make sure that at the halfway point, you're not far from fifty seconds into the lap. (Keeping your pace as even as possible will help you run your best times.)

This is just about all you need to know to fit right in on the track! When the specific workouts are explained in chapter 9, I'll explain how long to run and rest and what to do while you're resting (for the most part, a slow jog is best in between work intervals).

In the meantime, here's a simple track workout to try once you're comfortable with running a few miles: after running a one-mile warm-up at Easy pace, run half a mile (800 meters) at a fast pace, about the pace you could maintain for a mile or so. Time how long it takes you do it and then rest for that same amount of time by lightly jogging or even walking. Repeat four times, or for as many times as you find that you can maintain your initial 800-meter pace, before finishing with a one-mile cool-down at Easy pace.

FARTLEKS: AN ALTERNATIVE TO THE TRACK

If you don't feel like doing your speed work at the track—a lot of people think running around in a circle is boring, and I get that—there are other options. The simplest alternative is called a *fartlek* (no giggling!), a Swedish word meaning "speed play." To do a fartlek workout, you simply run along your normal route, but alternate periods of Easy running with short bursts of increased (but by no means breakneck) speed, often your 5K or 10K pace.

In a typical fartlek workout, you'd run at your Easy pace for five to ten minutes as a warm-up, then alternate, say, one minute of 5K pace running with two or three minutes of Easy running, repeating this "one minute at 5K pace, two to three minutes at Easy pace" sequence six times before switching back to pure Easy pace for a five-minute cool-down. Because the terrain will vary, and it's not as easy to measure distance on the roads or the trail as it is on the track, it will be harder to precisely gauge how your speed is improving and to consistently reach the same peak intensity with each workout. That's completely fine—it's called speed *play* for a reason! Have fun with it and don't get too caught up in exact paces for your fartlek workouts.

Speed work is tough, and it's something you'll probably want to do only once a week at first. The next type of workout is slightly less intense, but longer in duration.

Threshold (Tempo) Training

Your anaerobic threshold is the intensity at which your body transitions from a comfortable, aerobic state of exercise (where your Easy-pace runs should be) to the more stressful, demanding anaerobic state, in which your cells do not have sufficient oxygen to convert sugar into energy and you quickly fatigue as lactic acid builds up in your muscles. Threshold training (used interchangably with the term "tempo") teaches your body to increase the intensity at which your body transitions between the two types of activity—in short, it trains you to stay in "comfortable" mode longer and at higher speeds.

Threshold training is often described as "comfortably difficult": it should be an intensity that you can maintain for about forty-five to sixty minutes and no longer. If you've run a 5K recently, try a slightly slower per-mile pace than that one for your threshold training. You should be able to speak in short sentences while you're running at threshold pace, but getting a whole paragraph out should be tough. (As an example, if you can run a 5K in twenty-five minutes, try a threshold pace of around 8:30 minutes per mile.)

Start with twenty minutes or so at this pace and build from there to run faster and longer as your fitness improves. Work in some hills, or even do this run on a trail to keep it interesting, but you'll have to slow your pace to account for the rougher terrain.

The Long Run

The bread and (almond) butter of a distance runner's regimen is the long run. It's the longest workout of the week, and if you're training for your first half or full marathon, this is where you'll often run farther than you've ever run up to that point, making the long run an often anxiety-provoking workout, but also an extremely fulfilling one, once you have a chance to put your feet up and look at what you accomplished.

The long run isn't complicated; essentially, you run at Easy pace, one that's slow enough that you could easily carry on a conversation throughout the run. The low intensity required to complete the long run without leaving your body completely broken down means that the first half or more of the long run is usually quite comfortable, before the physical and mental effects of running for one, two, three, or more hours start to become very noticeable.

The hardest thing about the long run, in my experience, is the monotony. If you find that you get bored, you can break it up by bringing along an MP3 player loaded with a playlist, some podcasts, or even an audiobook if that's your thing. Just be careful to make sure you remain aware of what's going on around you, especially if you're running on roads.

If you're the outdoorsy type, you'll find that trail running is often far more exciting than running on roads and offers an escape from the busy world and a chance to meditate, think, or just relax while you do your long run.

The long run is the one where you'll need to make stops for water and nutrition (or bring it along with you), as described later in the chapter.

For the most part, you'll do your long runs at an Easy pace that you can maintain without too much effort until the final miles of the run. This is especially important the first time you train for a race to limit the risk of injury, but when training to improve on a previous time, consider several variations on the long run. You won't find any of these long run variations in the training plans in this book, but they're worth experimenting with as you gain experience.

The *progressive* long run involves gradually increasing your pace, so that even though you start out at Easy pace, by the end of the run you're doing something close to (if not faster than) your goal race pace. Similar ways to boost the aerobic benefit of the long run are to aim to "negative-split" the run, meaning, to run the second half of the workout faster than you do the first half, or run up a long, gradual hill for the final fifteen to twenty minutes of your run.

You might also find it useful to increase the pace of your entire long run over the default Easy pace. You've got to be careful here because you run the risk of doing more harm than good if you run your long run at too hard a pace, but if you have a time goal, one way to get faster is to do your long runs at closer to race pace than the normal Easy pace, which is one to two minutes slower than race pace. For example, in my training to qualify for the Boston Marathon, I ran several twenty-milers at speeds ranging from eight minutes per mile (forty-five seconds per mile slower than my 7:15 goal pace) down to 7:30 per mile (just fifteen seconds slower per mile than goal pace). This was the first time I had ever done long runs with paces so close to marathon pace, and they certainly helped to give me a level of familiarity with what race day would feel like when it finally came.

One more common way to vary the long run is to put a tempo run in the middle of it. A twelve-mile run could become a three mile warm-up, a six-mile tempo run, and a three-mile cool-down. This is a tough workout, challenging your lungs, your legs, and your head, so don't try it at the end of an already hard training week. But if for some reason you've had to miss a mid-week workout and you're looking for an added challenge in the long run, you might think about giving the combination long run/tempo run a try.

RUN DIRTY! TRAIL RUNNING BASICS

Why start trail running, when the roads are treating you just fine, thanks?

Running like a wild man or woman through the woods nurtures the soul. Trail running satisfies a primal need for movement through nature, presumably left over from our days as hunters. When things spin out of control in an age of iPads and Androids, running in the woods is one thing we can count on to be pretty much the same as it's always been.

That's your fancy explanation. My real reason for trail running? Getting dirty makes me feel *way* more badass than I am.

What else does the average road runner have to gain from venturing out into the wilderness?

Two things. First, reduced risk of injury: The soft, variable surface of the trail lessens the likelihood of an overuse injury, strengthens core muscles, and ultimately makes for more comfortable long runs than asphalt. Second, a rush that road running just can't give you. It should come as no surprise that soaking in the essence of the forest results in a quantifiably greater endorphin release than breathing in roadside fumes.

Trail running has done more than make me a stronger, happier runner—it has made me a runner, period. For seven years before finding the courage and initiative to learn a new type of running, I ran strictly on roads. I relished the day-to-day routine of my training, but I refused to call myself a runner until I could truly enjoy the act of running for its own sake. It took trail running to make me feel like a runner.

Here's what you need to know to hit the trails safely and discover this wildly soothing side of running.

Trail Running Gear

At its best, trail running is a more minimalistic endeavor than road running. Though audio players, GPS devices, and heart rate monitors have become musts for many runners, technology tends to take away from experience of trail running. Even a watch is dispensable.

Still, there are certain necessities for trail running, some of which require different considerations from running on roads.

- **Clothing:** The same technical apparel that you wear on roads works for trails, but choose something that you don't mind getting dirty or snagged.

- **Shoes:** Road shoes work fine for short runs. If you decide to stick with trail running, however, you'll eventually want to get a pair of trail shoes. They offer a stronger, more protective sole and greater stability than most road shoes. And although the idea of barefoot running on trails is appealing, it's smart to run a trail in shoes first to get a feel for how sharp those rocks are.

- **Water bottle:** If you're not big on drinking from streams, you're going to have to carry your water with you. A favorite among trail runners is the handheld water bottle that straps to the hand and has additional pouches for things like keys, ID, and food.

- **Insect repellent:** Depending on where you're running, bug spray may or may not be necessary.

- **Headlamp or flashlight:** One of the coolest things about trail running is that you can do it pretty safely at night without having to worry about cars. But for running at night, a headlamp or flashlight is absolutely necessary. The LED versions are both lightweight and bright.

And don't forget a towel and change of clothes, socks, and shoes for afterward. If you're doing it right, you'll be wet and dirty by the end of the run.

Seven Steps to Your First Trail Run

1. Find a trail. By far, the best way to start trail running is to find a local group of trail junkies and run with them. They'll know the best trails in your area and help you get started. I met my trail-running group through my town's running club; you can search for running clubs near you at Run the Planet's club directory: www.runtheplanet.com/resources/clubs.

If you can't find a group, the American Trail Running Association's website offers a free directory of U.S. and international trails: www.trailrunner.com/trails/main_international_page.htm.

(continued)

Distinguish between technical and non-technical trails. Non-technical trails are paved, gravel, or dirt roads that are generally easy to negotiate. Technical trails are narrow dirt or rocky paths offering every variety of challenge that most people associate with trail running.

2. Slow down and take short, quick strides. You can expect to run about 20 percent slower on trails for a given level of exertion than you would on roads. You'll find steeper hills, more side-to-side movement, and lots of obstacles to deal with. Trail running is most fun when you forget about pace and do what feels good.

Shorten your stride so that your weight is over your feet most of the time; this allows you to react quickly and maintain balance. You'll find that trail running works your core and stabilizer muscles more than road running, so it may help to focus on keeping your core engaged.

3. Don't be afraid to walk the hills. The surest way to identify a road runner on the trails is to look for the guy or girl who runs past everybody up hills, only to be passed again going downhill. Trail runners know that it's usually more efficient to walk up the steep hills and conserve energy to make up time on the way down.

4. Scan the ground five to ten feet in front of you as you run. When you're running trails, you need to pay extra attention to where you step. But you certainly don't want to be staring straight down at your feet the whole time.

Continuously scan the ground a few yards ahead of you while you're running. As you notice an approaching obstacle, shift your attention to your feet to do whatever is necessary to clear the obstacle. And don't be lazy—pick up your feet just a little higher than you think is necessary to avoid a root or rock. Too many falls happen because of complacency.

5. Keep a distance of ten feet from other runners. If you're going to pay attention to the ground in front of you, it helps if you can actually see it. If that's not enough reason to keep your distance, trail runners must change speeds all the time, rarely with warning. Nobody likes getting rear-ended.

6. Watch out for slippery roots and rocks. If you can step over a fallen tree, root, or large rock, rather than on it, do it. Lots of them are more slippery than they look. And when crossing streams, it's often safer to walk directly through the water than to try to tiptoe across wet rocks. (You'll avoid being called names, too.) It's trail running; you're supposed to get muddy and wet!

7. Be safe. It's not called "the wild" for nothing. You know, this is the common-sense stuff. Whenever possible, run with a friend. Bring a map if you're running a new trail for the first time. Have a first aid kit in the car and carry extra food for emergencies. Bring along a cell phone or pepper spray if you're running alone.

And know the area you're running—how to deal with the wildlife, when and where hunting takes place, when the sun goes down, and anything else that might pose a danger. You have everything you need—don't wait another day to hit the trails!

EVOLVING HAPPILY AS A PLANT-BASED RUNNER

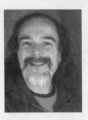

By Greg Watkins

I was 6-feet 1-inch tall and 180 pounds when I graduated high school. By age 20, I was morbidly obese.

I ate to excess my whole life, abused alcohol from my first drink, and lived in reckless disregard of everyone and everything. By the time I was 33 I was tipping the scales at more than 330 pounds. I developed several health problems including spinal damage, high blood pressure, pre-diabetes, and severe sleep issues. My lifestyle soon led to legal trouble as well. I got sober while awaiting trial but quickly began replacing alcohol with food. I was well on my way to eating myself to death, even as a vegetarian.

While incarcerated, I learned to do more with less. My diet was limited and controlled, but I was able to remain vegetarian. Movement and exercise were also controlled so I ran every chance I got. I learned that discipline was the real key to success and, oddly enough, freedom. Over three years I lost 160 pounds, became medication- and diabetes-free, and learned to love running.

I quickly began to have my doubts. I struggled with self-image and self-worth. And I struggled with my new body and the fact that it did not fix my mental and emotional self. I decided to enter a 5K and although that race caused me to fall in love with racing, it again failed to fix me.

Over the next couple of years I struggled with staying committed to running. Running wasn't working for me but neither was not running. Thankfully, something had changed in me. It was the nagging idea that running had saved my life, that I must run to live. I finally took stock of my situation and got honest with myself. I was back up to 210 pounds and was really unhappy with the way I looked and felt. I had been lazy in my training and careless in my nutrition. I was letting myself down, and I was responsible for the outcome. It was time to start looking for answers.

While running a local half marathon I saw a woman in a No Meat Athlete shirt. I looked up the website and it was like the missing piece fell into place. Just seeing a forum of other vegetarian athletes muddling through, not just arriving, was awe-inspiring. I read *Born to Run* by Christopher McDougall because of the NMA review, and I fell in love with the *idea* of running all over again. I ran for 59 days straight following Matt Frazier's example and fell in love with the *act* of running all over again.

Over the past year I have learned so much and been given so many gifts. I have learned to love running again and not to take myself too seriously. I have posted personal records at 5K, 10K, half marathon, and marathon distances. I have strengthened my resolve to continue my vegetarian lifestyle with designs on becoming vegan. I have been reminded that life is not about the destinations but the journey and wisdom is in the doing, not in the thinking. I will continue to challenge myself, not as penitence but for the growth and experience. I am committed to evolving happily.

How Cross-Training Can Help Your Running

There's a lot of argument about whether cross-training (engaging in exercise other than running) is beneficial, simply a waste of time, or worst of all, harmful for those whose goal it is to improve as distance runners. The benefits of cross-training, as I see them, are twofold:

▶ Cross-training allows you to work out and improve your overall fitness while giving your running muscles (and mind) a break; lower-impact or even zero-impact activities, like swimming and cycling, are often a welcome change from the pounding of roads and trails.

▶ Cross-training, particularly strength training, allows you to target certain muscles more effectively than running does and thus build a balanced body that's more resistant to injury than if you strictly ran.

Critics, on the other hand, point out that many elite marathoners don't cross-train. If your goal is to improve as a runner, they say, why put valuable training time into any other activity?

For the purposes of this book, let's put that criticism to bed. First and foremost, if you're new to fitness in general or inspired to get back in shape after years without exercise, I want you to do the activities you find most enjoyable. If you want to run, but not exclusively, and your goal is to improve your fitness more than it is to run your fastest race, by all means trade in a running workout for a serious swim in the pool, a bike ride, or a basketball game now and then. You'll stick with a lifestyle that you enjoy, and I don't want to tell you not to partake in those other activities, especially if your body hasn't allowed you to do so in a very long time.

Even for those who do want to focus exclusively on running goals, I'm a believer that cross-training can help all but the most genetically gifted of athletes. Many elite runners are elite because their bodies are built for running; they can put in hundreds of miles a week without breaking down. Most of us, no matter how disciplined and dedicated, simply will never get to that point without injury ruining the party.

That said, cross-training should play a limited role. Specifically, all else being equal and when your body can handle it, you should prefer to get in a quality running workout over a cross-training workout.

There are three primary instances where I think cross-training is beneficial to runners, discussed here in decreasing order of importance.

1. Light strength training, when done before or after running workouts, promotes strength and flexibility that will improve running efficiency and help prevent injury.

USA Track and Field-certified running coach Jason Fitzgerald addresses this subject on our advanced marathon training website, *Run Your BQ* (www.runyourbq.com):

> Before you can run twenty miles comfortably (or race a marathon well), you need to first be a good athlete. Overall strength, flexibility, balance, and coordination are essential even for marathoners. Weight routines in the gym and body weight exercises that can be done at home are one way to get more athletic.

Note that Jason said, "race a marathon well." If all you want to do is finish this one marathon in your lifetime before you put this silly running thing to bed, well, you can probably get by without strength training. But even then, a properly designed at-home routine of just five to ten minutes per day could significantly reduce your chances of getting injured during training and help you to make it not just to the start line, but across the finish line as well.

It's beyond the scope of this book, unfortunately, to provide detailed strength-training workouts, but I highly recommend you check out the Core Performance website (www.coreperformance.com) and series of books, specifically *Core Performance Endurance*, which was the first serious strength program I incorporated into my marathon training (and which essentially wiped out the nagging injury problems I still dealt with when I tried to train for marathons).

2. Low-intensity aerobic training, done in place of Easy runs, can help prevent mental burnout or allow you to maintain aerobic gains while limiting running mileage to recover from or prevent injury.

I'm a huge proponent of the Easy run in-between tougher running workouts. I've experimented with the approach of replacing it entirely with cross-training, as suggested in certain low-mileage training plans that have recently become popular, but I actually found myself *more* susceptible to injury when I didn't have those easy miles to log in between workouts. Just as importantly, I realized how much I needed them mentally, when the same amount of time and effort in a pool or on a bike just didn't have the same meditative effect that easy running does for me. (As the saying goes, "I run because it's cheaper than therapy.")

But I do see the benefit of long, slow, cross-training workouts as a replacement for the occasional Easy run. There are times in any training program when your legs feel like they need a break, and you get the strong sense that even your Easy run will do more harm than good. When you just can't justify taking the day off, a light cross-training workout can serve you well. If you enjoy swimming, cycling, cross-country skiing, or any other endurance sport, this is the time to work it into your training schedule. Just keep in mind that what you have scheduled is an Easy run, so make sure you keep your cross-training at that same easy, conversational pace.

3. Higher-intensity endurance training can serve as a temporary replacement for quality running workouts while you allow an injury to heal.

Finally, I can see one main time for high-intensity (as supposed to easy) cross-training: when you're injured or seriously worried about an injury that's coming on. You may still want to get in a high-quality workout, and if you know for sure that your cross-training workout won't aggravate the injury that you're supposed to be allowing to heal, then go for it.

SHOULD YOU BOTHER TO STRETCH?

Many runners stretch religiously before and after their runs, often for no other reason than because it's what they see other runners doing. And everyone knows, from as far back as gym class, that stretching prevents injury. Right?

Not so fast. In fact, the truth could be just the opposite. Traditional, static stretching before a workout (meaning no movement, as opposed to dynamic stretching) may actually increase the likelihood of injury by reducing running economy, maximal power, and strength before your workout even begins. Additionally, stretching a cold muscle (i.e., one that hasn't been warmed up) is a great way to invite a pull or strain.

But certainly, flexibility is an asset to a runner, as is a light warm-up before a workout. If you're choosy with your strength training exercises, you'll increase flexibility with them, but you can simultaneously achieve both aims of increasing flexibility and raising your body temperature and heart rate through dynamic stretching, a form of stretching that involves movements not entirely unlike those you perform while running.

You'll find several such routines in the book *Core Performance Endurance,* and *Runner's World* details a free dynamic stretching routine which you can find at their website: www.runnersworld.com/stretching/dynamic-routine.

Fueling Before, During, and After Your Workouts

Of all the meals you'll eat during your training, those surrounding your workouts are the most crucial to your success, particularly because they affect your ability to recover in time for the next workout. Fortunately, the precepts of optimal workout nutrition are completely consistent with plant-based nutrition. In fact, vegan ultramarathon legend Scott Jurek once pointed out that most people eat a plant-based diet anyway while they're running.

However, the food that will maximize performance and recovery differs significantly from what you should eat as part of your normal diet—most noticeably, the focus shifts toward simple, sugary carbohydrates. The reason is simple; most of the time, you want your body to have to work a little to break down the food you take in. But a workout is one time when you want the opposite: easily-digestible, quick energy sources.

The following guidelines will help you to ensure that you're taking in adequate nutrition to power your workouts—before, during, and after.

A Pre-Workout Nutrition Primer

1. Consume carbohydrates and protein in a 3:1 ratio. The 3:1 ratio is almost universally advocated for optimal absorption of nutrients before a workout. For a big workout, it's best to eat a large meal three to four hours ahead of time, so that your stomach can be completely rid of the food by the time you start moving, and then eat a small snack of mostly carbohydrate (say, a banana or a few dates) just before the workout begins.

The less time you have until your workout, the smaller your "large" meal should be: if you've got an hour or more, thirty grams of carbs and ten grams of protein is great; otherwise, halve the amounts. Mark Verstegen of Athletes Performance Institute recommends a scoop of protein powder in about six ounces (175 ml) of Gatorade or watered-down orange juice. I've found this little pre-workout drink to be easy and convenient when I don't have a lot of time between when I'm eating and my workout.

If you choose to include fat in your pre-workout meal (which can help with nutrient absorption) do so only in moderation because fat takes longer to convert to energy during physical activity than carbohydrate and causes gastrointestinal distress in some people. Five grams of fat should be plenty for this purpose.

2. Include quick-working, high-glycemic carbs for energy now, sustained release (but not necessarily starchy) carbs for energy later. For example, if you're making your own pre-workout drink, you might use dates (glucose) as the high-GI, instant-energy sugar, and agave nectar (fructose) for slower energy release, like *Thrive* author Brendan Brazier does in many of his concoctions.

Why no starchy bagels or bread? To convert starch into usable sugar requires your body to work, and during a workout, you'd like to use your available energy for movement, not digestion. This guideline applies mainly to workouts that last up to three hours. For longer workouts and events, the intensity becomes low enough that it's not a problem to consume and digest starchier foods, and you'll likely find yourself craving them.

3. Get a head start on electrolyte replacement. Lack of electrolytes can do more than just bring on a nasty bonk; in fact, it's downright dangerous. Hyponatremia is the condition of having too much water and not enough sodium (an electrolyte) in your system, and it has proved fatal for endurance athletes who load up on water but don't replace electrolytes that are lost during physical activity.

Lots of electrolytes are lost through sweat, and you should take in salt and other electrolytes during your workout to replace them. Coconut water and most sports drinks and gels contain electrolytes, so you'll get them during your workout if you're consuming any of those drinks. But you can get a head start on electrolyte replacement simply by adding ¼ teaspoon of salt, which contains 500 to 600 mg sodium, to your pre-workout drink.

CARBOHYDRATES: SUSTAINABLE FUEL FOR MILES AND MILES

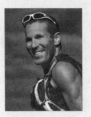

By Adam Chase
Team Salomon ultrarunner and adventure racer, Running Times *Trail and Gear Editor*

I became a vegetarian 30 years ago when I was a waiter at a country inn that served a lot of bacon and sausage. Seeing these products cook on cookie sheets was enough to make me decide not to ingest them, and this choice quickly spread to all meat and then dairy, eggs, and seafood.

When I was traveling and racing internationally, I added a limited amount of dairy, mostly in the form of cheese, back into my diet as a way of getting protein when plant-sourced alternatives weren't readily available. The best example of this was during the four-day long Raid World Championships in Argentina and Chile, where beef was the primary source of calories and almost the sole source of protein, so a little cheese went a long way.

I mostly eat carbohydrates and the vast majority of those come in the form of various dry breakfast cereals, consisting of whole grains, oats, dried fruits—what my friends jokingly call "twigs and rabbit food." I've been feeding or grazing off of a big freezer bag mix of whole-grain cereals that I eat at my desk for much of the morning after a run and before a mid-afternoon workout for more than 20 years now, and it never seems to get old.

Carbs make for great fuel for me. They sustain me and are sustainable. They taste good and go down easy. They burn clean and are about as convenient as you can get. And the fact that no animal suffered in their production certainly sits well with me, too.

Eating and Drinking during Your Workout

For short workouts (less than forty-five minutes), a quick pre-workout meal will get the job done and carry you through the workout. But for any workout lasting longer than that, or in very hot conditions, you'll want to replace lost fluid and electrolytes and replenish carbohydrate stores during the workout. Here's how to choose what (and how much) food and drink you take in while you're on the move.

1. Consume mostly liquids or easily-digesting food. Solid food takes more energy and blood to digest than liquid, leaving you with less for running. And solid food is more likely to cause intestinal distress, which can ruin a workout or race.

Energy gels are designed to be easy to digest and to pack a lot of carbohydrates (plus electrolytes) into a small space. Amazingly, nature created a food with those exact same properties—dates! Most of the time, I bring along a handful of fresh, whole dates instead of energy gel because I prefer the taste and texture (they're more like gummies than gel) and I like the idea of fueling with whole food over processed. Just don't forget to remove the pits!

If you're a gel person, I suggest making your own, especially if, like me, you're not a fan of the taste or makeup of most commercial varieties. See my recipe for homemade energy gel on page 111.

Energy gels are designed to be easy to digest and to pack a lot of carbohydrates into a small space. Amazingly, nature created a food with those exact same properties—dates!

2. Take in four to six ounces (120 to 175 ml) of water every ten to twenty minutes. Your goal is to replace most of what you lose in weight, so if you want to get precise, you can figure out what you lose during a standard workout and drink the exact amount you need to replace it. But for all but the most serious athletes, that level of precision is unnecessary, and a rule of thumb like this one suffices.

3. Get 500 milligrams of sodium with every sixteen ounces (475 ml) you drink. As mentioned above, when you sweat, you lose electrolytes, and that puts you at risk for hyponatremia if you hydrate without replacing them. If you're making your own drinks and gels, 500 milligrams is about the amount in ¼ teaspoon of salt (this will vary slightly depending on the type of salt you use).

4. For workouts and races lasting longer than an hour, you need thirty to sixty grams of carbohydrate per hour. If your workout is shorter than an hour, you probably don't need to take in any calories during it, and your main nutritional concern is hydration if you'll sweat a lot. But if you'll go beyond forty-five minutes, it doesn't hurt to have a little something, either in liquid or solid form, to help you stay strong at the end.

Thirty to sixty grams per hour is the standard recommendation, and if you prefer to think in terms of calories, aim for 120 to 250 calories per hour, mostly carbohydrates. These are big ranges, as your true needs will vary according to a whole host of factors. With awareness and experience, you'll be able to narrow the range to one that works best for you. For a more precise starting point, divide your body weight in pounds by four to determine your minimum hourly carbohydrate requirement in grams. Some experts say that a little bit of protein as well, in a 4:1 carb-to-protein ratio, helps minimize muscle damage.

For mid-length workouts, up to two hours, my preferred sources of carbohydrates are sports drinks, dates, or a combination of the two. Bananas and other soft fruits are great, too. For lower-intensity workouts that last longer than two hours, you may find you want something besides sugar; I like to bring along a pita with hummus or almond butter, pretzels, and other convenient, starchy, salty foods on long runs.

Maximize Recovery with Proper Post-Workout Nutrition

Every athlete can appreciate the joy of the post-workout meal. It's a celebration of a job well done, and the food we eat when a long workout has left us ravenously hungry usually tastes better than any other. Fortunately, eating immediately after a workout serves us by jumpstarting the recovery process. When you chow down post-workout, follow the guidelines below to choose food that will make the most of the work you've done to earn it.

1. Respect the recovery window. In the fifteen to forty-five minutes immediately following a workout, your muscles are primed to receive fuel to start the repair process. Eat (or drink) your recovery meal right away, within the first half hour after the workout, to begin the recovery process.

2. Make your immediate post-workout meal easy to digest. Your muscles need blood to deliver nutrients to them. The more of that blood that's tied up in digesting a solid food, the less that gets to your muscles. Ideally, you should get your immediate post-workout fix in liquid form, like a smoothie or shake.

3. Consume 0.75 grams of carbohydrate per pound of body weight and include protein in a 4:1 or 5:1 carb-to-protein ratio. I'm not usually one for specific numbers when it comes to food, but these are so common that I had to list them. Your carbohydrates should include high-glycemic index carbs, like glucose (again, dates are great), and some slower-release carbohydrates as well. And don't forget the fat—include about half as many grams of healthy fat as you do protein. Several of the energy bar recipes in this book have appropriate nutrient ratios to make them perfect for a post-workout snack.

4. Drink 2 cups (475 ml) of water per pound of body weight lost during exercise. Do I really expect you to weigh yourself after each workout and drink a corresponding amount of water to make up for it? Of course not. But if you have access to an accurate scale, you can weigh yourself after a typical workout to get an idea of how much water you need, then use that as a guideline for future workouts. Easier, I think, is just to drink a few cups (475 to 700 ml) of water immediately after the workout and more throughout the day until your urine is nearly clear.

5. Replace lost electrolytes. Hopefully you've done this before and during your workout, but you'll want to take in electrolytes once more to help with recovery. Some good sources of electrolytes are fruit, coconut water, dulse flakes, a few pinches of sea salt, and Nuun tablets.

And remember: Recovery doesn't stop with your post-workout meal. You'll want to eat again an hour or two later, this time focusing more on quality protein. After your long runs, you'll probably find that you get hungry frequently throughout the day, as often as every two hours or so. This hunger is a message from your body that it needs food to replace the calories you burned and rebuild your muscles for the next workout, so don't ignore that message.

NEVER RUN ON EMPTY

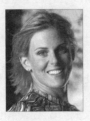

By Hillary Biscay
Ironman triathlon champion, Ultraman World Championship finisher
www.hillarybiscay.com

My primary concern with fueling pre- and post-workout is simply never going empty—before or afterward. Even before an early morning swim or run, I always take in some calories. For me, proactive fueling is the name of the game so I always try to eat enough that I don't end up feeling starving or low on energy mid-workout.

The amount of calories and timing of fueling pre-workout depends on what I am doing. If it's running, I like to give myself a good 45 minutes between eating and exercise, and I keep the food simple, most likely some gluten-free and vegan toast with peanut butter and jam. If I am swimming, I can pretty much shove anything into my mouth up to the minute I start the session and be fine. Still, my rule across the board is to avoid getting full, because for me, full equals lethargic.

After a training session of any substance, I aim to get in calories and hydration in the "fueling window," or within 20 minutes or so of finishing. My go-to post-workout fuel is a Vega protein shake; these shakes are essential to my daily nutrition because they provide me with high-quality, complete vegan protein from hemp, brown rice, and peas. I blend these shakes up in my Vita-mix with frozen fruit, greens, and veggies to help me recover and get some of my essential nutrients for the day.

CHAPTER 9

TRAINING FOR YOUR FIRST (OR YOUR FASTEST) RACE

Of the millions out there who call themselves runners, only a small contingent runs solely for running's sake. These runners don't train for races or fitness or any other external motivator like these—instead, they run to run. Because they need it. Because they live for it.

I deeply admire runners like this. And I wish I could call myself one of them. But in fact, I didn't even consider myself a "real" runner until after I qualified for the Boston Marathon in my sixth marathon. This isn't because I thought that beating a certain time was necessary to enter the sacred community of runners; in fact, I don't think speed or ability has anything to do with the "runner" label. Instead, it's about mindset: I didn't come to love running until I had experienced all that it took for me to accomplish a goal like qualifying for Boston.

How did I get myself to work so hard at the goal if I didn't love running itself? Simple: it wasn't the act of running that energized me—instead, it was the process of training. There's a big difference.

As I wrote in the introduction, it was the decision to run a marathon that got me started with running. I had never run more than three or four miles at a time before I made the decision that I would become a marathoner, so marathon training was my first real experience with running. In that way, training—not for some undefined goal in the future, but for a specific goal on a specific day—was all I knew of running. And that process of being diligent, of being driven, and of preparing is what I fell in love with.

A few years back, Starbucks used to print inspirational quotes on its coffee cups. I feel a bit sheepish spouting coffee-cup wisdom, but one quote from an author that I read on my cup of *grande* bold has stuck with me:

The irony of commitment is that it's deeply liberating—in work, in play, in love. The act frees you from the tyranny of your internal critic, from the fear that likes to dress itself up and parade around as rational hesitation. To commit is to remove your head as the barrier to your life.

—Anne Morriss

Training for a race requires commitment. It requires a sense of discipline; it means getting out of bed or out the door at a set time on set days—sometimes when it's cold, sometimes when it's raining, and sometimes when you'd just rather roll over and hit the snooze button or grab a seat on the couch and a glass of wine and call it a day.

> *Those days I mentioned, when running is the last thing you feel like doing, are the days when sucking it up and making it happen will benefit you the most*

I've taken a valuable lesson from training as a runner: Those days I mentioned, when running is the last thing you feel like doing, are the days when sucking it up and making it happen will benefit you the most. The endorphins will start flowing, and you'll come home energized (you might even feel like extending your run!). In other words, what seems the hardest in the moment is often what you most need.

And when you do accomplish that victory, rather than giving into the moment's temptation to ease up, nothing feels better than marking that "X" on your schedule or recording your run in your journal or wherever you keep track of your workouts. You battled the urge to slack off, you got out there, and you beat it. Today, you put in the work. Now get some rest, because it won't be long until it's time to do it all again.

FROM COUCH POTATO TO IRONMAN—IN TWENTY MONTHS

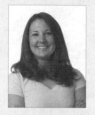

By Susan Lacke
No Meat Athlete *resident triathlete,* Competitor *magazine columnist, Ironman, and semi-professional cupcake eater*

"Anyone can do an Ironman. Anyone."

I was giving a friend a massage after he completed his twelfth Ironman triathlon—a race that consists of a 2.4-mile swim, 112-mile bike run, and 26.2-mile run—when he uttered those words.

"Pssht. Susan, it's nothing. Anyone can do an Ironman. Anyone. Really, it's not that big of a deal."

I had just run my first 5K a few months prior. Before that, I was a couch potato who was trying to quit smoking (again). Ironman triathlons were something crazy people did.

Call it a runner's high. Call it temporary insanity.

Anyone can do an Ironman? Anyone?

Count me in.

From 5K to Ironman

When I signed up for that first 5K, I assumed I'd run the 5K, cross the accomplishment off my bucket list, and go back to being a couch potato. But that didn't happen.

If you sit on the sidelines of an Ironman finisher's chute long enough, you'll believe that anyone can run an Ironman too. There's such a wide cross-section of Ironman triathletes, from chiseled studs to eighty-year-old nuns. After sitting at enough finish chutes, I decided I didn't want to be a spectator anymore. I wanted to know what it was like to be on the other side.

The next time I saw an Ironman finisher's chute—just twenty months after making the resolution to run a 5K—I was running down it.

(continued)

Nine Keys to Preparing for Your First Ironman

It was a series of bold choices, hasty mistakes, happy accidents, and finally, focused planning that took me from couch potato to Ironman in just twenty months. Everyone has their own way of doing things when it comes to Ironman, and when you train for one, you'll discover yours. For now, here are what I found to be the nine most important keys in going from zero to Ironman faster than most people think is possible.

1. Start small. Don't make Ironman your first goal. Start small and then gradually build from there.

My initial goal, in 2009, was to run a 5K. The race was so much fun I wanted to run another one—so I did! I spent an entire summer running 5K races before deciding to make a jump to the half marathon distance that fall.

As part of my half marathon training plan, I started doing some cross-training—a little swimming here, a little mountain biking there, a few weights there—and all the while, had fun and enjoyed my new hobby.

2. Choose a race and commit to it. If you're thinking about doing it, stop.Plenty of people think. They have dreams and ambitions and goals, and they're beautiful, but you need to become a person who stops thinking and starts doing.

If you want to do an Ironman, the first step is the most important one: Pick a race and commit to it. Nothing lights a fire under your ass like the email confirming your registration for an Ironman—and the $500-plus receipt that comes with it.

3. Find those in the know. No one expects you to be an expert in triathlon before beginning your training for Ironman. But what is expected is that you'll be willing to seek out those experts.

Instead of trying to decipher tri-speak on my own, I asked for help—a Masters Swim group, a running group, triathlete and cyclist friends, my local triathlon shop, and every book and article I could find on Ironman training.

I spent just as many, if not more, hours learning about Ironman than I did actually training for the Ironman itself.

4. Progress one small step at a time. Focus on the next race weeks away, not on the Ironman months away.

It took me a while to learn, but when you focus on the training that needs to be done for the sprint, then the Olympic distance, then the half-Ironman, then the full Ironman, you gradually build your distance in a way that won't overload you, burn you out, or have you peaking too early.

Ironman is the big picture, but it's made up of a lot of little brushstrokes. Focus on the brushstrokes.

5. Make lots of mistakes—and learn from each one. You will make mistakes—lots of them and too many to count. Anyone who says they didn't make at least one mistake while training for an Ironman is a liar. Mistakes happen. It's the people who are willing to admit and learn from those mistakes who truly succeed in moving past them.

I ignored friends who told me I was doing too much, too soon. They warned of burnout, and I certainly experienced it—to the point where one of my friends came over to ride with me one morning, and I was in bed, crying.

"Please don't make me get on my bike today," I begged. Finally, I understood what my friends meant by "burnout."

I would skip rest days, feeling like those were a luxury I couldn't afford. I only had a short amount of time to prepare, I worried, and every second wasted resting was a second which could have been spent getting stronger. I was given a mantra to repeat every night: "You get faster when you rest." It became a meditative phrase, keeping me in check when I felt antsy.

I focused too much on the physical nature of training and not enough on mental focus. I learned both are equally important.

I made mistakes in refueling after workouts until I finally realized that good post-workout food made it so much easier to get up the next day for another training day. I made tweaks to my diet, many of them based on *Thrive* author Brendan Brazier's advice.

6. Aim for balance, not sacrifice. Ironman training is time-consuming, yes. But it doesn't have to negatively impact your work, family time, or social life—it's about finding the right balance.

While training for my first Ironman, I moved from Wisconsin to Arizona; balanced a full-time job, part-time teaching, and part-time writing; worked on my doctoral program; maintained my social ties; and somehow still managed to live a balanced life.

It wasn't always easy. I'd often wake up at four o'clock in the morning to get my training done before work, and sometimes I had to skip or cut short a workout so I could meet a deadline instead. I was known for skipping out on happy hour in favor of an eight o'clock bedtime, but everyone also knew

(continued)

I'd make it up to them by taking them out for a post-ride brunch on Sunday. I knew my priorities and constantly sought to maintain balance.

7. Have a support system. Having people to support you goes hand-in-hand with finding balance. A support system of people will know when to say "Quit being a baby!" and when to say "Oh, you poor baby!" They'll understand why you fall asleep during the afternoon matinée and will happily give up their French fries when you ask, "Are you gonna eat all those?" They'll smile when you have a good training day and give you a hug when you have a bad one.

And when you finally do run down that finisher's chute, they will cheer louder than anyone there. In a way, it's their big day, too!

8. Go forward with blinders on. I hate the word impossible–hate it, hate it, hate it.

Anyone who does an Ironman needs to learn to hate that word, too. You'll hear it during your training, and it'll sneak into your thoughts after a bad run or when you panic during your first open-water swim start.

"Impossible" is your mind's way of tricking your body into quitting. "Impossible" is what you say when you're too scared to keep trying. "Impossible" is the easy way out when you begin to doubt yourself.

Fear and self-doubt can be powerful, but the only way to overcome them is to face them head-on.

I won't lie: I had a lot of "oh, *bleep*" moments, especially in the days before the race. But I also had a lot of really good people who were able to talk me down before I gave up altogether (see #7).

9. Enjoy every second of it. Most people sign up for one Ironman, finish it, and then rack their bike in the garage, never to be ridden again.

I'm not that person. I love this sport and have continued to train and race since finishing that first Ironman. Triathlon has given me the best health of my life, a group a friends who are like family, and a sense of accomplishment with each workout completed and each finish line crossed.

If there's one thing I learned going from couch potato to Ironman in twenty months, it's that twenty months can change a lot. And I enjoyed every single second of it. I still do.

I don't mean to oversimplify the sport. It's work. It's dedication and commitment and perseverance. But it's still fun. I wouldn't do this sport if it wasn't.

Is It for You?

Many people train for much longer than twenty months before even thinking about registering for their first Ironman. My path just happened to be a little shorter. It's not the path for everyone, but it worked for me.

I still stand by my assertion that anyone can do an Ironman. It's just that most people won't.

Don't get me wrong—the sidelines of an Ironman finisher's chute are pretty cool. But actually being in the finisher's chute? You'll never understand what it's like until you find out for yourself.

About the Four Training Plans

In this chapter, you'll find four different training plans. They range from a basic plan for running your first 5K (starting with just about zero running experience) to a plan for running a fast half marathon, with many tough workouts along the way to increase your speed and endurance and improve your overall fitness. These plans were developed with the help of Jason Fitzgerald, a 2:39 marathoner, USA Track and Field–certified coach, and author of the uber-informative and inspiring blog Strength Running (www.strengthrunning.com). Jason is also the co-creator and running mastermind behind Run Your BQ (www.runyourbq. com), a comprehensive resource and community he and I developed with one goal: to help our dedicated, passionate members qualify for the Boston Marathon. The plans in this chapter are as follows:

1. A 5K plan

2. A 10K plan

3a. A half marathon plan for those who want only to finish

3b. A half marathon plan for those who want to gain serious fitness or run a fast time

The Workouts

The training plans make use of many different workouts, each designed with a specific purpose in preparing you for your race. For reference, each workout is explained in detail below, so that when it shows up in your plan, you'll know exactly what to do.

Easy: Easy miles (described in more detail in chapter 7) should be exactly that. The purpose of Easy running is to build your aerobic base with only the most minimal stress on your body while you recover from the previous workout. You should be able to easily carry on a conversation during your Easy run. If you'd like a more objective measure of the intensity, use a heart rate monitor and keep your heart rate below 70 percent of your maximum heart rate.

Most people run their Easy miles too hard. Easy pace should feel *really* slow. If you're worried about running into someone you know for fear that they'll make fun of you, you're probably doing Easy pace just right.

Easy miles appear simply as numbers on the training schedules without a specified workout type.

Fartlek (10K plan only): A fartlek is most easily described as a short duration of relatively fast running. The description is intentionally vague—after all, it means *speed play*, so we don't want to be too strict about the exact pace. Here, the only fartlek paces we suggest are your 5K and 10K paces. Don't worry about running at exactly those paces; just increase your intensity so that you're approximating how you'd run in a race of that distance. For example, if your workout says "4 miles: 6 x 1 minute Fartlek @ 5K pace, 90 seconds Easy jog in between," here's what you'd do that day:

Warm up with Easy-pace running for three to five minutes. Speed up to your 5K pace for one minute (having fun, of course!) and then do ninety seconds of Easy pace jogging before increasing again to 5K pace. Repeat the "1 minute of 5K pace followed by 90 seconds of Easy jogging" for a total of six times. Then do Easy pace jogging for as far as you need to go to bring your total mileage to the day to four miles.

Notice that the fartleks usually will not take up the entire mileage for the day (in this example, four miles). In general, any fast running should be done in the middle of your run, preceded and followed by periods of Easy running to reach the day's total mileage goal.

Interval A: A "repeat" in this workout is defined as running relatively hard for one minute and then running at Easy pace (or walking, if necessary to fully recover) for two minutes.

"Running relatively hard" does not mean sprinting, but speaking full sentences at this pace should be difficult. Your pace should be just slightly slower than the fastest pace you could smoothly maintain for the entire work interval. (It may take you a workout or two before you find the right pace that allows you to complete the workout.)

After a five-minute Easy-pace warm-up, do six repeats, followed by a five-minute Easy-pace cooldown. If, after any work interval, you do not recover to the point of being able to easily carry on a conversation before it's time to start the next, perform the cooldown and end the workout.

Interval B: This is the same as Interval A, but each repeat is now 1:30 (1 minute, 30 seconds) of hard running followed by 2:30 of Easy recovery.

Tempo A: After a five-minute warm-up, run two miles at a "comfortably hard" intensity. This should be significantly harder than Easy-pace, but not so hard that you have trouble speaking in full sentences. (Tempo pace should be around thirty seconds per mile slower than your 5K race pace.) Finish with a five-minute cooldown.

Tempo B: This is the same as Tempo A, but after a five-minute warm-up, run three miles, followed by the five-minute cooldown.

Hill A: On a moderately-sloped hill that takes about three minutes to run up, run up the hill at an intensity somewhere between Tempo intensity and Interval intensity—a good indicator is that while you should be able to speak in short sentences, a conversation or even long sentences would be difficult while running up the hill. (Note that though the intensity you feel here should be greater than what you feel during a Tempo run, your actual speed will probably be slower because of the hill.)

Don't get hung up on the details: The exact grade of the hill doesn't matter, nor does the exact intensity. The point of this workout is simply to get your body accustomed to running on hills and give you a more productive workout than Easy pace does.

Once you've reached the top of the hill, turn around and jog slowly and comfortably back down (this should take you the same amount of time or slightly longer than it took to run up the hill). Up-and-down counts as one repeat.

After a five-minute Easy-pace warm-up, do two repeats, followed by a five-minute Easy-pace cooldown. If, after any work interval, you do not recover to the point of being able to easily carry on a conversation before it's time to start the next, perform the cooldown and end the workout.

Hill B: This is the same intensity as Hill A, but choose a hill that takes four minutes to run up and perform an additional repeat, for a total of three repeats between the warm-up and cooldown.

Long: The long run each week should be done at a very low intensity (the same as Easy), one to two minutes slower per mile than you're capable of running the distance. Just as with Easy runs, aim to be able to carry on a conversation without difficulty during long runs.

Cross-Train: Cross-training workouts can be any physical activity you like other than running, performed at a moderate intensity for anywhere from a few minutes up to about forty-five minutes. Running is not recommended on these days, as the point is to give your running muscles and joints a break while still allowing you to improve your fitness. Recommended cross-training activities include cycling, spinning, swimming, light strength-training (go easy on the legs), pilates, yoga, dance, etc. Read more about cross-training in chapter 8.

Foam Roll: Foam-rolling on the day after your long run (or as often as you like throughout the week) is an optional activity aimed at softening brittle muscles and speeding recovery. By rolling muscles back and forth across a dense foam roll or, in some cases, a tennis ball, you simulate a myofacial-release massage that helps prevent injury by relaxing and loosening tight, brittle muscles, in addition to stimulating blood flow for the recovery process. Like a deep massage, foam rolling is a bit uncomfortable at first, but after a few sessions, it begins to feel great. It also requires minimal financial investment—you can pick up a foam roll for less than $20. See www.nomeatathlete.com/foam-rolling for a sample foam roll routine.

How to Use These Training Plans

Although you can use these plans individually, they're designed to fit together as a progression. The 5K plan assumes that you can run for one or two minutes without stopping at the outset; it will train you to run for a continuous 3.1 miles. The 10K plan starts at three miles and gets up to seven miles at its longest (slightly more than a 10K), serving as a bridge between the 5K plan and a half marathon program. And either half marathon plan, of course, will take you to the finish line of your first 13.1-mile race.

What's the point? In about nine months' time, with the habit-forming techniques described in chapters 2 and 7 and a commitment to put the work in, it's not at all unreasonable to think that you could go from couch potato to half marathoner. I get emails all the time from ecstatic new runners who have done just that, in well under a year's time. Of course, the one-after-another approach won't be for everyone. Many readers will have already run a 5K, for example, and will want to jump right into the 10K plan or even the half marathon plan. Both of these options are feasible, and I've included a bonus "base-building" plan to help you build your mileage a bit before you start either.

Each plan describes exactly what Jason Fitzgerald and I recommend you do on each particular day. To get started, simply choose a target race and count backward on a calendar to figure out when you need to begin your official training schedule. Below each plan are notes that elaborate on the terminology and workouts in the given plan. Don't skip these! They contain critical explanations that will clear up confusion and make sure you're using the plans as intended.

"DO I HAVE TO TRAIN FOR A 10K IN-BETWEEN MY 5K AND HALF MARATHON?"

It's also entirely reasonable (though it requires more caution to avoid injury) to complete the 5K plan in this chapter and then jump right into half marathon training, skipping the 10K race or incorporating one into your training. In this case, I'd recommend using the base-building plan before you start half marathon training to help you increase your weekly mileage from the 5K program's peak up to what's needed before starting the half marathon plan.

What to Do if You Need to Miss a Workout

There's something about having a training schedule laid out in front of you and specifying exactly what to do each day that makes you (or at least, it makes me) want to follow it to the letter—to be disciplined, to be meticulous, and to never miss a single workout.

As hard as it may be to do, I urge you to let go of the tendency to strive for perfection. That may run counter to most of the "aim high, shoot for the stars" achievement advice you'll hear, but there's a good reason for it.

The most important thing to focus on as you go through the ups and downs of training is your ultimate goal. For me, and, I suspect, most others, the goal is none other than the race itself. Sure, overall health and fitness and the confidence and fulfillment that result are all underlying motivators, but in the day-to-day routine of following a training program, it's that prize—race day—at the end of the schedule that gets you out the door to train.

This goal, then, is where you'll look in moments of uncertainty about the proper course of action. Having the race as your most important goal dictates that, should an injury or even just some excess fatigue force you to decide between completing a scheduled workout or skipping it, the deciding factor should be which course of action maximizes your chances of making race day a success.

View These Training Plans as Roadmaps

At www.nomeatathlete.com, I offer in-depth guides for completing your first marathon and half marathon on a vegetarian or vegan diet. They're called, respectively, the *Marathon Roadmap* and *Half Marathon Roadmap*.

That word, "roadmap," is a perfect analogy to illustrate the idea of letting your ultimate destination dictate your actions along the way.

Imagine you're embarking on a cross-country road trip, say, from New York City to Los Angeles, and you want to get there reasonably quickly. At the outset, you (or your GPS) have a particular route in mind. It's the best route, the one that, if all goes according to plan, will get you there the fastest with the least amount of wear and tear on your car, maximizing your chances of making it without a breakdown.

It'd be nice if things worked out perfectly, and you were able to stick to your planned route from start to finish. But with 3,000 miles to cover, it's a certainty that you're going to hit a snag somewhere along the way that will call for an adjustment.

At some point, a road will be closed for construction. Another time, you'll approach the beltway of a major city right at rush hour. In neither case is it in your best interest to blindly follow your map without a detour. If your only goal were perfect execution of the route without deviating one iota, what would you do? Well, you'd plow right through the construction zone and drive straight into rush hour—both of which would reduce your chances of making it across the country with your car in one piece and without having a breakdown (nervous or automotive).

But following the ideal route to the letter isn't the goal. The goal is to make it across the country. You realize that your ideal route was just that—an ideal, not one that you had much hope of following perfectly. When it serves you and your ultimate goal to do so, you let yourself veer off course a little bit. You'll find your way back to your route, of course, but you'll need to make a few adjustments to get back on track in the smartest possible way. For example, rather than driving right back to where you left off after a detour, you realize you can cut some miles off the journey by meeting up with your route at the next major city.

All of this has a close (hopefully obvious) analogy to your training, with the ultimate destination of our hypothetical road trip representing your race.

As you increase your training mileage and push beyond your comfort zone to grow, you're going to deal with aches, pains, and possibly even more serious injuries. The advice on running form and the training principles in this book will do everything possible to keep you healthy, but it's a fact of running that a decent percentage of runners get hurt (that figure is often quoted as high as 60 or 70 percent per year).

What happens when something doesn't feel right or when your body is telling you that you need a break? Answer: you take that break.

How to Adjust the Training Plans When You Need To

As you gain experience as a runner, you'll learn which aches and pains are routine for you and which ones signal something potentially more serious. When you decide it's in your best interest to skip a workout, don't hesitate to do so. Remember, your goal is to complete your race and do well in it—it is *not* to complete every workout in a program that you committed to before you had any information about how your body would respond to the stresses of training! In light of new information that your hip is bothering you or something is wacky with your IT band, the correct course is no longer the initial, best-case training plan.

If you have reason to believe that an injury is imminent, take an unplanned day off or replace a scheduled hard workout with an easy run, cross training, or a day of rest and foam rolling. If you need to, rearrange the week's workouts to give yourself consecutive days off.

If you have reason to believe that an injury is imminent, take an unplanned day off.

And if you have the sense that your long run on the weekend is going to do more harm than good—and that's really the key consideration—then skip it. Or, because my beginning half marathon plans have you reducing your long-run distance after several weeks of increase, replace the scheduled long run with a shorter one if that seems more reasonable and then make up the long one next week if you're feeling better.

Also, my half marathon and marathon plans always include a taper period, which includes a weekend or two of reduced-mileage long runs leading up to race weekend. Tapering allows you to arrive at the race feeling fresh, but an additional reason to build in taper time is to add some flexibility to the runner's schedule: it allows you to shift your entire training plan back by a week, in the case that injury, fatigue from overtraining, mental burnout, or simply life's manner of getting in the way force you to miss a key workout or even take an entire week off of training.

Finally, there's the question of whether you should try to make up missed workouts. My answer is that it depends. If you miss an Easy run or cross-training day, don't worry about making it up. Enjoy the day off and join back up with your plan the next day. If you miss a tougher workout, but not a long run, you might try to make it up, but only if your schedule can easily accommodate it.

For example, let's say you're training for a half marathon, using the Fitness plan, and because of severe weather or some other reason, you need to miss your Thursday hill workout. Should you try to do it on Friday? Well, you've got a long run coming up on Saturday, and it's not a good idea to do the hill workout and long run in back-to-back days. But if your schedule allows you to push your long run back to Sunday, then you could do it. Run your hill workout on Friday, rest on Saturday, run long on Sunday, then take the scheduled recovery day on Monday and resume the plan with Tuesday's speed workout.

Our goal isn't to have you complete every workout; it's to have you cross the finish line of your race and have a good time doing it.

If your schedule isn't so friendly and pushing your Saturday long run back to Sunday isn't an option, then don't worry about the missed hill workout. It's water under the bridge—trying to cram it in would mean back-to-back tough workouts, and if you try to do that (especially if your reason for skipping the workout in the first place was injury-related), you'll lose more than you gain.

The moral of this long section, in short, is this: these training plans are flexible. Our goal in designing them isn't to have you complete every workout; it's to have you cross the finish line of your race and have a good time doing it. Sometimes, that will mean rearranging the plan or skipping workouts entirely, and that's absolutely not something you should feel any guilt about. Come race day, a single workout (or even a few workouts) won't make a hoot of difference.

NO MEAT
ATHLETE

WHAT IT TAKES TO BECOME A VEGAN BODYBUILDER

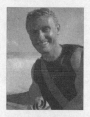

By Robert Cheeke

Author and Founder of Vegan Bodybuilding & Fitness,
www.veganbodybuilding.com

In the fall of 1999, I made the unconventional decision to set aside my athletic strength to pursue an athletic weakness. I had completed one season of NCAA collegiate cross country running for Oregon State University, but lifting weights and the sport of bodybuilding tugged at my heart.

To illustrate how foreign weight lifting and bodybuilding were to me at the time, consider that I became vegan as a 120-pound fifteen-year-old, and at the time of my change in athletic pursuit, I was a 155-pound nineteen-year-old devoted to running. Weight training was seemingly not my thing—I thought running was. Nonetheless, in an effort to achieve greater happiness, I hung up my running shoes and replaced them with weight lifting gloves.

How do you succeed in this kind of transformation, one that requires a whole new lifestyle and set of demands on the body? Here are the steps I took:

- Determine specific goals and be as detailed as possible. Include concrete timelines, identify the meaning behind the goals, and create a plan.

- Be consistent with nutrition and training. Consistency leads to adaptation, improvement, and success. You can't get to point C without going through points A and B first.

- Learn from those who have been there before. The changes in your nutrition and training programs are best left to trainers, teachers, or mentors who have advice based on first-hand experience. It's not just about eating more and training more. It's about eating right and training smart.

- Don't expect results overnight. If you're new to lifting weights, your body is likely to respond faster than someone who has been weight training for

(continued)

a while. At the same time, you need to cultivate a measure of patience to ensure success over the long term.

- Be realistic. I'm the first person to encourage others to dream big and pursue their passion, but don't think that after a year or two of weight lifting you'll look like the people in muscle magazines. Understand that the body has limitations and work within them, naturally and drug-free. But work hard and dream big anyway.

- Don't buy into the hype. We all know bodybuilders and weight lifters need to consume more protein than chess players. But don't get sucked into the idea that you have to go out and buy a bunch of supplements, pills, powders, and packages of "vegan meats" to achieve your muscle-building goals. Eating whole foods in adequate quantities with proper ratios of carbohydrates, proteins, and fats is the most nutritionally sound method to fuel your body. Fruits, vegetables, legumes, nuts, grains, and seeds will be your fuel sources.

- Document your meal plans and workouts. Having a record to reflect back on will help in the assessment of your progress or lack thereof. Without a record, you won't really know what you're really doing from day to day.

- Continue to educate yourself. Study anatomy and physiology to learn how the body works. When you understand how muscles, joints, and the nervous system function and the role food plays as fuel, you become a smarter athlete.

- Take a break. Your muscles need rest to repair and grow. Not allowing proper recovery time can result in, at best, exhaustion and a lack of wellness, and at worst, torn and damaged muscles that leave you sidelined for weeks or months, unable to progress. I find five days of weight training a week to be enough for optimum results.

- Have fun. If weight training isn't fun at least most of the time, it's time to find something else to do. You never know what activity might resonate with you. As long as you're pushing yourself hard in any form of fitness on a regular basis, you are likely building a stronger body.

I followed those ten steps during a bodybuilding career that spanned a full decade. The time came just recently to ask myself the same question I posed at the beginning; would the pursuit of something else make me happier? I answered that question a few months ago, and as fate would have it, I put my running shoes back on.

If You Want to Go Farther. . .

Unfortunately, space and scope considerations kept me from including marathon and ultramarathon training plans in this book. Marathon training (and beyond) is serious business, in that it requires a bigger commitment and affects your lifestyle more than even half marathon training does. For that reason, I'd be doing you a disservice to include those training plans and give you the idea that with just a simple plan, eighteen weeks from now, you'll be tearing up your first 26.2.

For marathon training, invest in a more comprehensive program than a simple schedule. Don't get a free plan that you randomly find online; get a book and make a more serious study of the ins and outs of training. Decide what's important to you in a marathon training program and look for one that matches your needs—is it a "just finish" plan? A "break four hours" plan? A low-mileage program? One that includes a lot of cross-training and will groom you for (one day) Ironman training? Or perhaps it's a program that focuses on diet, strength training, and other fitness goals (weight loss, for example). Chances are there's a plan out there that fits the bill.

I've mentioned my own marathon training program, *Marathon Roadmap,* and its half marathon counterpart. This isn't the place for a sales pitch, but I feel compelled to mention it because it's a book written for those who want to run their first marathon on a plant-based diet—whether it's someone who has run a marathon before and is new to veganism, or a longtime vegetarian or vegan who has just recently been bitten by the marathon bug. You can learn more at my website: www.nomeatathlete.com/resources.

For the shorter distances—5K, 10K, and even half marathon—you have all you need (half marathon training is a big enough commitment that I decided it deserved its own book for those who wanted to go more in depth, but the information in the book you're holding is more than sufficient to help you cross the finish line).

With that, you're ready. If you've made it this far, you have all the running know-how you need. Now it's a matter of putting it into action, if you haven't already. For myself and so many others, action starts with a compelling goal and a strong "why" behind it, so it's my hope that as you've read this book, you've crystallized in your mind a vision of what's possible—and that the information and training programs here will help you make that vision a reality.

Training Plan for Your First 5K

Using the following chart as your guide, alternate running and walking for the indicated durations until you complete the distance specified in each workout. Use the stopwatch function on your watch so that you know when it's time to switch between the two. For example, the first workout says "1 mile: Run 1 minute, walk 1 minute." This means to begin your workout by running for a minute, then walk for a minute, then run for a minute and then walk for a minute, until you have covered a total of one mile.

All running in this plan should be at Easy pace. Walking should be brisk but comfortable, a distinctly slower pace than your Easy running pace, so that you can recover in time to run again.

Although you'll get up to three miles at a time as early as Week 8 in this plan, note that these early three-milers involve intervals of walking and are therefore easier than your 5K race will be. Don't be intimidated when you see "3 miles" on the schedule!

This plan is flexible! The actual days of the week are not important; you can shift the schedule around as needed. But keep a day of recovery (or active recovery, in the form of cross-training) between any two runs.

Week	Active Recovery Sunday	Recovery Monday	Base Run Tuesday	Active Recovery Wednesday	Base Run Thursday	Recovery Friday	Long Run Saturday
1	Cross-train and/or foam-roll	Rest	1 mile: Run 1 minute, walk 1 minute	Cross-train	1 mile: Run 1 minute, walk 1 minute	Rest	1 mile: Run 2 minutes, walk 1 minute
2	Cross-train and/or foam-roll	Rest	1 mile: Run 2 minutes, walk 1 minute	Cross-train	1 mile: Run 1 minute, walk 1 minute	Rest	1 mile: Run 2 minutes, walk 1 minute
3	Cross-train and/or foam-roll	Rest	1 mile: Run 3 minutes, walk 30 seconds	Cross-train	1 mile: Run 1 minute, walk 1 minute	Rest	2 miles: Run 2 minutes, walk 1 minute
4	Cross-train and/or foam-roll	Rest	2 miles: Run 3 minutes, walk 30 seconds	Cross-train	1.5 miles: Run 1 minute, walk 1 minute	Rest	2 miles: Run 4 minutes, walk 1 minute
5	Cross-train and/or foam-roll	Rest	2 miles: Run 4 minutes, walk 30 seconds	Cross-train	1.5 miles: Run 2 minutes, walk 1 minute	Rest	2 miles: Run 6 minutes, walk 1 minute
6	Cross-train and/or foam-roll	Rest	2 miles: Run 5 minutes, walk 30 seconds	Cross-train	2 miles: Run 2 minutes, walk 1 minute	Rest	2.5 miles: Run 6 minutes, walk 30 seconds
7	Cross-train and/or foam-roll	Rest	2.5 miles: Run 6 minutes, walk 30 seconds	Cross-train	2 miles: Run 2 minutes, walk 1 minute	Rest	2.5 miles: Run 8 minutes, walk 30 seconds
8	Cross-train and/or foam-roll	Rest	2.5 miles: Run 8 minutes, walk 30 seconds	Cross-train	2.5 miles: Run 2 minutes, walk 1 minute	Rest	3 miles: Run 10 minutes, walk 30 seconds
9	Cross-train and/or foam-roll	Rest	2.5 miles: Run 8 minutes, walk 30 seconds	Cross-train	2.5 miles: Run 2 minutes, walk 1 minute	Rest	3 miles: Run 12 minutes, walk 30 seconds
10	Cross-train and/or foam-roll	Rest	2 miles: Run 10 minutes, walk 1 minute	Cross-train	1 mile: Run entire distance	Rest	5K race

Training Plan for a 10K

Except for specified fartlek workouts, all mileage in this plan should be at Easy pace. This plan is flexible—the actual days of the week are not important; you can shift the schedule around as needed. But keep a day of recovery (or active recovery, in the form of cross-training) between any two runs.

Mileage without a specified workout is to be done at Easy pace. Consult the Workout section on page 222 for instructions about each type of workout. Note that the long-run milage in Week 3 actually exceeds 10K—this is okay since you'll be running at much slower than race pace in order to build comfort at longer distances.

	Active Recovery	Recovery	Fartlek Workout	Active Recovery	Base Run	Recovery	Long Run
Week	Sunday	Monday	Tuesday	Wednesday	Thursday	Friday	Saturday
1	Cross-train and/or foam-roll	Rest	3 miles: 6x1 minute Fartlek @ Goal 10K pace, 2 minutes Easy jog in between	Cross-train	2 miles	Rest	4 miles
2	Cross-train and/or foam-roll	Rest	3 miles: 8x1 minute Fartlek @ goal 10K pace, 2 minutes Easy jog in between	Cross-train	2 miles	Rest	4 miles
3	Cross-train and/or foam-roll	Rest	4 miles: 8x1 minute Fartlek @ goal 10K pace, 2 minutes Easy jog in between	Cross-train	2 miles	Rest	5 miles
4	Cross-train and/or foam-roll	Rest	4 miles: 8x90 seconds Fartlek @ goal 10K pace, 2 minutes Easy jog in between	Cross-train	2 miles	Rest	5 miles
5	Cross-train and/or foam-roll	Rest	3 miles: 8x1 minute Fartlek @ goal 10K pace, 2 minutes Easy jog in between	Cross-train	4 miles	Rest	5 miles
6	Cross-train and/or foam-roll	2 miles	5 miles: 8x1 minute Fartlek @ 5K pace, 2 minutes Easy jog in between	Cross-train	5 miles	Rest	6 miles

NO MEAT ATHLETE

7	Cross-train and/or foam-roll	2 miles	5 miles: 8x1 minute Fartlek @ 5K pace, 2 minutes Easy jog in between	Cross-train	5 miles	Rest	6 miles
8	Cross-train and/or foam-roll	3 miles	5 miles: 8x90 seconds Fartlek @ 5K pace, 90 seconds Easy jog in between	Cross-train	5 miles	Rest	7 miles
9	Cross-train and/or foam-roll	Rest	4 miles: 8x90 seconds Fartlek @ 5K pace, 90 seconds Easy jog in between	Cross-train	4 miles	Rest	5 miles
10	Cross-train and/or foam-roll	Rest	4 miles: 6x1 minute Fartlek @ 5K pace, 90 seconds Easy jog in between	Rest	3 miles	Rest	(Optional warmup: 5 to 10 minutes Easy running) 10K Race!

Half Marathon Training Plans

The two half marathon plans, while indicating similar total mileages each week, differ in their difficulty. The "To Finish" plan is the lowest-risk plan, in the sense that if your goal is to finish a half marathon and no more, this is the most likely plan to get you there. It also happens to be the simpler of the two, focusing on Easy-paced mileage rather than incorporating speed, hill, and tempo workouts.

The tougher but more rewarding workouts, around which the "Fitness" plan is built, will help you not only finish your half marathon, but do so in style—and by that, I mean you'll be fitter and faster than if you had done the "To Finish" workouts instead. Of course, these rewards come at additional risk: although every effort has been taken to injury-proof these plans as much as possible, the simple fact remains that running harder will more likely result in injury than will putting in consistent, gentle, conversational miles. Which plan you choose is up to you—let your current fitness level and the goal that truly energizes you be the deciding factors.

Both programs start with roughly twelve total miles in the first week and increase from there. If you're not yet at that level, you'll need to first build your mileage base for several weeks.

If you can't yet run a 5K (3.1 miles): The first step is to get up to 5K distance because most of the workouts in these programs are three miles or more in length. If you can't run a 5K yet, I suggest you use the 5K program in this chapter to train for a race of that distance before moving on to either 10K or half marathon training.

If you can run a 5K, but you're not comfortable running several of them in one week: The first thing to recognize, in this case, is that most of your training miles (especially if you're following the "To Finish" plan) are run at a pace significantly slower than your 5K race pace. Keep in mind that an easy-paced three-mile run will be much easier on your body than a "raced" 5K.

Still, you may find you have more confidence if you complete the 10K program here first. That will take you, over the course of ten weeks, from being able to run three miles to being able to run six or seven, and from there, you'll be in an excellent position to start half marathon training.

It's not necessary to have run a 10K before you start training for a half marathon. But if you choose to go right from 5K to half marathon, and you haven't been running anywhere near 12 miles per week, you'll need to build up a stronger mileage base before you start the program.

For example, a six-week base-building schedule, to be done after you've run a 5K but *before* Week 1 of either of the half marathon plans here, might look like this:

	Active Recovery	Base Run	Base Run	Recovery	Base Run	Recovery	Long Run
Week	**Sunday**	**Monday**	**Tuesday**	**Wednesday**	**Thursday**	**Friday**	**Saturday**
1	Cross-train and/or foam-roll	2 miles	1 mile	Rest	2 miles	Rest	3 miles
2	Cross-train and/or foam-roll	2 miles	1.5 miles	Rest	2 miles	Rest	3 miles
3	Cross-train and/or foam-roll	2 miles	2 miles	Rest	2 miles	Rest	3 miles
4	Cross-train and/or foam-roll	2 miles	2.5 miles	Rest	2 miles	Rest	3 miles
5	Cross-train and/or foam-roll	2 miles	3 miles	Rest	2 miles	Rest	3 miles
6	Cross-train and/or foam-roll	2.5 miles	3 miles	Rest	2.5 miles	Rest	3 miles

NO MEAT ATHLETE

Here, all numbers represent Easy mileage. This base-building period starts at only eight miles per week, assuming you're comfortable running three miles once a week, and adds mileage at less than 10 percent per week until total weekly mileage reaches eleven miles. After completing this six-week period, you could begin Week 1 of the "To Finish" following plan, and the weekly workout schedule would remain consistent in terms of days of the week.

Even for someone who can already run a 5K, there's nothing wrong with taking more than six weeks to build your aerobic base before you begin your official twelve-week training program. For example, if you haven't been running eight miles per week (which the above base-building schedule calls for in Week 1), add lower-mileage weeks to the beginning of the schedule. If, as another example, you reach the end of the base-building schedule and the mileage feels difficult, repeat the final week (assuming it's not overly strenuous) until you're comfortable increasing your mileage and beginning the official twelve-week half marathon program.

The "To Finish" and "Fitness" Plans

For each of the two following plans, when no workout type is specified and only a number appears, that number represents Easy-pace miles, except for Saturdays, when it represents Long run mileage. See the Workouts section on page 222 for descriptions of all the workout types (Long, Easy, Tempo, Hill, and Interval).

The actual days of the week are not important. Feel free to shift the schedule according to what day works best for you. For example, if you'd prefer to do your long runs on Sundays rather than Saturdays, simply shift the schedule by one day to accommodate this. But try to keep the order of rest days and workouts roughly the same.

The Wednesday workout each week is an option of either a cross-training workout or a complete rest day, depending on which you feel you'll benefit most from at that point in the program. If you're not sore, fatigued, or otherwise in need of a day off, I'd recommend doing some light cross-training here.

Weeks 4 and 8 are reduced-mileage weeks designed to give your body a chance to rest and recover. It is not recommended that you do more than is specified in these weeks.

The mileage of the two plans is very similar; they differ mainly in workout intensity and variety. On a given day, you can do the corresponding workout from the opposite plan if you need a break (if you're doing the "Fitness" plan) or are up for a tougher workout (if you're following the "To Finish" plan).

In all workout descriptions in the Workouts section, the warm-up and cool down should be easy running, at the same conversational pace as Easy workouts. If desired, you can do some light dynamic stretching or other activity to raise your heart rate before or after the workout.

The "To Finish" Plan

Week	Active Recovery Sunday	Base Run Monday	Base Run Tuesday	Active Recovery Wednesday	Base Run Thursday	Recovery Friday	Long Run Saturday
1	Cross-train and/or foam-roll	2 miles	3 miles	Rest/cross-train	3 miles	Rest	4 miles
2	Cross-train and/or foam-roll	2 miles	3 miles	Rest/cross-train	3 miles	Rest	5 miles
3	Cross-train and/or foam-roll	2 miles	3 miles	Rest/cross-train	3 miles	Rest	6 miles
4	Cross-train and/or foam-roll	2 miles	3 miles	Rest/cross-train	3 miles	Rest	4 miles
5	Cross-train and/or foam-roll	2 miles	3 miles	Rest/cross-train	3 miles	Rest	7 miles
6	Cross-train and/or foam-roll	2 miles	3.5 miles	Rest/cross-train	3 miles	Rest	8 miles
7	Cross-train and/or foam-roll	2 miles	3.5 miles	Rest/cross-train	3 miles	Rest	9 miles
8	Cross-train and/or foam-roll	2 miles	4 miles	Rest/cross-train	3 miles	Rest	4 miles
9	Cross-train and/or foam-roll	2 miles	4 miles	Rest/cross-train	3 miles	Rest	10 miles
10	Cross-train and/or foam-roll	2 miles	4.5 miles	Rest/cross-train	3 miles	Rest	11 miles
11	Cross-train and/or foam-roll	2 miles	4.5 miles	Rest/cross-train	3 miles	Rest	5 miles
12	Cross-train and/or foam-roll	2 miles	3 miles	Rest	1 to 2 miles	Rest	Half marathon: 13.1 miles

The Fitness Plan

	Active Recovery	Base Run	Interval Workout	Active Recovery	Tempo/Hill Workout	Recovery	Long Run
Week	Sunday	Monday	Tuesday	Wednesday	Thursday	Friday	Saturday
1	Cross-train and/or foam-roll	2 miles	Interval A	Rest/cross-train	Tempo A	Rest	4 miles
2	Cross-train and/or foam-roll	2 miles	Interval A	Rest/cross-train	Hill A	Rest	5 miles
3	Cross-train and/or foam-roll	2 miles	Interval A	Rest/cross-train	Tempo A	Rest	6 miles
4	Cross-train and/or foam-roll	2 miles	Interval A	Rest/cross-train	Hill A	Rest	4 miles
5	Cross-train and/or foam-roll	2 miles	Interval A	Rest/cross-train	Tempo A	Rest	7 miles
6	Cross-train and/or foam-roll	3 miles	Interval B	Rest/cross train	Hill B	Rest	8 miles
7	Cross-train and/or foam-roll	3 miles	Interval B	Rest/cross-train	Tempo B	Rest	9 miles
8	Cross-train and/or foam-roll	3 miles	Interval A	Rest/cross-train	Hill A	Rest	4 miles
9	Cross-train and/or foam-roll	3 miles	Interval B	Rest/cross-train	Tempo B	Rest	10 miles
10	Cross-train and/or foam-roll	3 miles	Interval B	Rest/cross-train	Hill B	Rest	11 miles
11	Cross-train and/or foam-roll	3 miles	Interval B	Rest/cross-train	Tempo B	Rest	5 miles
12	Cross-train and/or foam-roll	3 miles	3 miles	Rest	1 to 2 miles	Rest	Half marathon: 13.1 miles

MORE ON THE FITNESS PLAN

Finally, in the fitness plan, make sure that the shorter workouts are not overly stressful on your body. They should be mildly difficult and invigorating, but recovering in time for the next run should not be an issue. If it is, lower the intensity at which you perform the shorter workouts or even replace them with Easy runs if that's what it takes to be ready for the next long run.

You Have Everything You Need. Now Make It Happen.

If you have made it this far and complete one of the training programs in this chapter, then have no fear: you're ready to race. By understanding the basics of running and nutrition outlined in this book, you're light years ahead of most beginning athletes lined up at the starting line for the first time in a 5K, 10K, or half marathon. And even if you haven't followed every habit-forming tip, nutrition guideline, and workout to the letter (hey, nobody's perfect!), you're likely more prepared than you realize.

Remember what I wrote earlier about setting goals, and how the real reason to strive for one is because of the person it will force you to become in the process? Keep that in the back of your mind as you progress. When things get tough or an injury sets you back, know that through the process of training, including eating a diet that's both wholesome and aligned with your values, you've steeled more than your body—you've undergone a transformation whose effects run far deeper than the physical.

Finally, enjoy every minute of the process of preparing and of the race itself. Marvel at and be grateful for your body, even when those last few miles really hurt and you have to dig deeper than you ever have before. You didn't choose to do this because you thought it would feel good 100 percent of the time, right? You're doing something incredible; relish that fact and enjoy every moment.

All that's left now is to trust your body and your mind, and make something awesome happen. I wish you the best of luck—be smart and go kick ass.

RESOURCES

This section is by no means intended to be a comprehensive listing of all the incredible resources available in the world of plant-based diets and fitness. Instead, my co-author Matt Ruscigno and I have narrowed our list by simply including some of the books, films, websites, and miscellaneous resources that we personally use, have used, or are involved with and recommend for fellow plant-based athletes. Some are obviously best for those who are new to a plant-based diet or even a healthy lifestyle, while others are valuable at any stage of your plant-based fitness journey.

Books

NUTRITION AND FOOD

The China Study by T. Colin Campbell

Chris Carmichael's Food for Fitness by Chris Carmichael

The Complete Idiot's Guide to Plant-Based Nutrition by Julieanna Hever

Disease-Proof Your Child by Joel Fuhrman

The Food Revolution by John Robbins

Food Rules: An Eater's Manual by Michael Pollan

In Defense of Food: An Eater's Manifesto by Michael Pollan

The Plant-Powered Diet by Sharon Palmer

Super Immunity by Joel Fuhrman

Thrive by Brendan Brazier

Vegan For Life by Jack Norris and Virginia Messina

Vegetarian Sports Nutrition by D. Enette Larson-Meyer

COOKBOOKS

1000 Vegan Recipes by Robin Robertson

*Anjum's New Indian** by Anjum Anand

Appetite for Reduction by Isa Chandra Moskowitz

Blissful Bites by Christy Morgan

Clean Food by Terry Walters

Jai Seed eCookbook by Julie Piatt and Rich Roll

Let Them Eat Vegan by Dreena Burton

Madhur Jaffrey's World Vegetarian by Madhur Jaffrey

Peas and Thank You by Sarah Matheny

*Rice and Curry: Sri Lankan Home Cooking** by S.H. Fernando Jr.

Simply Vegan by Debra Wasserman and Reed Mangels

Superfood Kitchen by Julie Morris

Thrive Foods by Brendan Brazier

Veganomicon by Isa Chandra Moskowitz and Terry Hope Romero

*Not an exclusively vegetarian cookbook, but contains several excellent vegetarian and vegan recipes.

FITNESS, RUNNING, OTHER SPORTS, AND INSPIRATION

The 4-Hour Body by Timothy Ferriss

Born to Run by Christopher McDougall

ChiRunning by Danny Dreyer and Katherine Dreyer

Core Performance Endurance by Mark Verstegen and Pete Williams

Daniels' Running Formula by Jack Daniels

Eat and Run by Scott Jurek

Finding Ultra by Rich Roll

The Power of Habit by Charles Duhigg

Relentless Forward Progress by Bryon Powell

Run Less, Run Faster by Bill Pierce, Scott Murr, and Ray Moss

Vegan Bodybuilding & Fitness by Robert Cheeke

THOUGHT-PROVOKING READS

Animal Liberation by Peter Singer

Eating Animals by Jonathan Safran Foer

I am a Strange Loop by Douglas Hofstadter

Why We Love Dogs, Eat Pigs, and Wear Cows: An Introduction to Carnism by Melanie Joy

Documentaries

Earthlings

Forks Over Knives

The Spirit of the Marathon

Unbreakable: The Western States 100

Vegucated

Blogs, Websites, and Magazines

VEGAN AND VEGETARIAN

7 Day Vegan (www.7dayvegan.com)

Choosing Raw (www.choosingraw.com)

Happy Cow (www.happycow.net)

No Meat Athlete (www.nomeatathlete.com)

Oh She Glows (www.ohsheglows.com)

PCRM's 21-Day Vegan Kickstart (www.pcrm.org/kickstartHome)

Post Punk Kitchen (www.theppk.com)

Thrive Forward (www.thriveforward.com)

True Love Health (www.truelovehealth.com)

Vegan Body Building & Fitness (www.veganbodybuilding.com)

Vegan Health and Fitness Magazine (www.vhfmag.com)

Vegetarian Nutrition (www.vegetariannutrition.net)

VegNews (www.vegnews.com)

Vegan Yack Attack (www.veganyackattack.com)

YumUniverse (www.yumuniverse.com)

SPORTS AND HABIT CHANGE
(Not Necessarily Plant-Based, Although Some Are)

Daily Mile (www.dailymile.com)

Good Form Running (www.goodformrunning.com)

iRunFar.com (www.irunfar.com)

Nerd Fitness (www.nerdfitness.com)

Rock Creek Runner (www.rockcreekrunner.com)

Runner's World Race Finder (www.runnersworld.com/race-finder)

stickK (www.stickk.com)

Strength Running (www.strengthrunning.com)

Zen Habits (www.zenhabits.net)

Training Resources and More from No Meat Athlete

No Meat Athlete Community and Forums (www.nomeatathlete.com/community-message-boards)

No Meat Athlete Half Marathon Roadmap: The Vegetarian Guide to Conquering Your First 13.1 (www.nomeatathlete.com/half-marathon-roadmap)

No Meat Athlete Marathon Roadmap: The Vegetarian Guide to Conquering Your First 26.2 (www.nomeatathlete.com/roadmap-system)

No Meat Athlete's official Facebook page (www.facebook.com/nomeatathlete)

No Meat Athlete's official Twitter page (www.twitter.com/nomeatathlete)

No Meat Athlete's Plant-Based Endurance Advantage E-course (www.nomeatathlete.com/plant-based-endurance)

Run Your BQ (www.runyourbq.com)

PCRM's VegRUN Program (www.vegrun.org)

Podcasts

No Meat Athlete Podcast (www.nomeathlete.com/category/radio-2)

The Rich Roll Podcast (www.richroll.com/category/podcast)

Ultrarunner Podcast (www.ultrarunnerpodcast.com)

Supplements, Food, and Miscellaneous

Brooks Running Shoes (www.brooksrunning.com) *— all Brooks running shoes (not their walking shoes) are vegan-friendly! Other shoe manufacturers, like New Balance, Luna, and Merrell, offer several vegan-friendly running shoe options, but for the most part it depends on the particular model. When in doubt, ask!*

Ezekiel Bread—*sprouted-grain breads*

Food Fight! Grocery (www.foodfightgrocery.com)—*all vegan store in Portland, Oregon, also does mail order*

Vega (www.myvega.com)—*natural, plant-based sports supplements*

Vegan Essentials (www.veganessentials.com)—*an online retailer with more than 1,200 all-vegan items in stock)*

ACKNOWLEDGMENTS

From Matt Frazier

Thank you to my mentors and inspirations, in writing, entrepreneurship, and (in several cases) veganism:

Seth Godin, Tony Robbins, Leo Babauta, and Tim Ferriss. What I've learned from you—not just what you teach, but the way you teach it—is the foundation for everything I do.

Sonia Simone, Brian Clark, Tony Clark, Jon Morrow, and everyone at Copyblogger Media. It's easy to look at *No Meat Athlete*'s history and pinpoint the exact moment when I started learning from you all, and to this day I continue to do so.

Caitlin Boyle, whose support in the early days of *No Meat Athlete* made all the difference.

Karol Gajda, Gena Hamshaw, and Robert Cheeke, without whose examples I might never have found the inspiration to become vegan. Brendan Brazier, Rich Roll, and Scott Jurek, the pinnacles of what's possible that I always like to point to, all three of you generous supporters of *No Meat Athlete* from early on. And Douglas Hofstadter and Richard Dawkins, the first to (very likely inadvertently) plant the seed in this one reader's head that maybe I didn't want to eat other thinking, feeling beings not all that different from me.

The *No Meat Athlete* team, who somehow make this operation seem halfway legit: Susan Lacke, Doug Hay, and Erin Frazier. We can get back to normal now.

Charlie Pabst, Bren Dendy, Jenny Leonard, Christine Hein, and Kevin McCarthy, all of whom have helped to make No Meat Athlete look sharp. Alright, cute.

The experts who contributed their collective wealth of knowledge to this book: Matt Ruscigno, Brendan Brazier, Jason Sellers, Christine Hein, Mo Ferris, Jason Fitzgerald, Robert Cheeke, Meredith Murphy, Ed Bauer, Erika Mitchener, Sara Beth Russert, Hillary Biscay, Adam Chase, Leo Babauta, Gena Hamshaw, Mike Zigomanis, and Susan Lacke.

The readers who were kind enough to share their stories to inspire others: Tina

Žigon, Pete DeCapite, Greg Watkins, Tom Giammalvo, Janet Oberholtzer, Tori Brook. Hearing stories like yours is the best part of this gig, bar none.

Recipe testers for this book: Tim Frazier, Vickie Craven, Christine Hein, Bren and Joe Dendy, Pete and Kristin DeCapite.

My family: Mom, Dad, Christine, Erin, Holden, and Ellarie. You're the reason for all of this.

Supporters of *No Meat Athlete* from day one: Colleen and Joel Baldwin and Pete and Kristin DeCapite.

Jamie Halberg, who helped me keep my head on straight throughout the daunting task of writing a "real" book.

Marcus Leaver, Cara Connors, Winnie Prentiss, Kevin Mulroy, and everyone at Fair Winds Press, for your help in making this project a reality and reaching far more people with this message than I could ever do on my own.

Last and most important, the *No Meat Athlete* audience, including but extending far beyond those who contributed photos for the inside covers of this book. Without you to support, share, interact with, and care about our work, No Meat Athlete would be a long-ago abandoned blog with a few recipes and a clever name—and I would still be a guy searching for something meaningful to do.

Thank you all. So much.

From Matthew Ruscigno

First and foremost I'd like to thank Matt Frazier for all the hard work he does and for involving me with this wonderful book. The team of editors we have worked with from Fair Winds Press have been helpful beyond belief.

Also my colleagues Reed Mangels, Ph.D., R.D., and Tim Radak, Dr.P.H., R.D., who answered technical questions for me, Ginny Messina, M.P.H., R.D., and Jack Norris, R.D., who have paved the way for this type of work and all of the volunteers at the Vegetarian Nutrition Dietary Practice Group of The Academy of Nutrition and Dietetics who continue to provide the science behind plant-based nutrition.

I'd also like to thank my professors at Loma Linda University who always challenged me to find the best research on vegetarian diets.

I am also very thankful for my early influences on living compassionately: Animal Defense League, Earth First!, Vegan Outreach, and Earth Crisis, to name just a few.

Last, my family, especially my mom and dad, and friends—there are too many of you to name—who have supported me throughout my entire life. No one person does anything alone—it's always with the support of friends and family. Thank you!

ABOUT THE AUTHORS

Matt Frazier is a vegan marathoner and ultrarunner as well as the founder of www.nomeatathlete.com, a 20,000+ subscriber blog about plant-based nutrition and fitness.

Matt started No Meat Athlete in 2009 when he decided for ethical reasons to become vegetarian, despite a concern that giving up meat would limit his ability to qualify for the Boston Marathon, a goal he had pursued for seven years. To his surprise, the change of diet had the opposite effect, and six months later, Matt qualified with a marathon time of 3:09:59, an improvement of more than 100 minutes over his first marathon time of 4:53. Within the next year, Matt ran two 50-mile trail ultramarathons, and he recently finished his first 100-mile race. He lives in the Western North Carolina mountain town of Asheville with his wife, son, daughter, and two rescued dogs. Follow him at www.nomeatathlete.com, @nomeatathlete on Twitter, and on Google+.

Matthew Ruscigno, M.P.H., R.D., holds two degrees in nutrition and is past chair of the Vegetarian Nutrition Dietary Practice Group of the Academy of Nutrition and Dietetics. In addition to his public health work, Matthew has a private practice and works closely with vegan athletes. An athlete himself, he has raced "The World's Toughest Iron-distance Triathlon" in Eidfjord, Norway, ultra-marathons, and 24-hour mountain bike races. He is a 3-time finisher of the Furnace Creek 508, a 500-mile non-stop bike race that National Geographic calls the 8th hardest race in the world. Matthew contributed to the bestseller *Appetite for Reduction: 125 Fast and Filling Low-Fat Vegan Recipes* by Isa Chandra Moskowitz.

NO MEAT
ATHLETE

INDEX

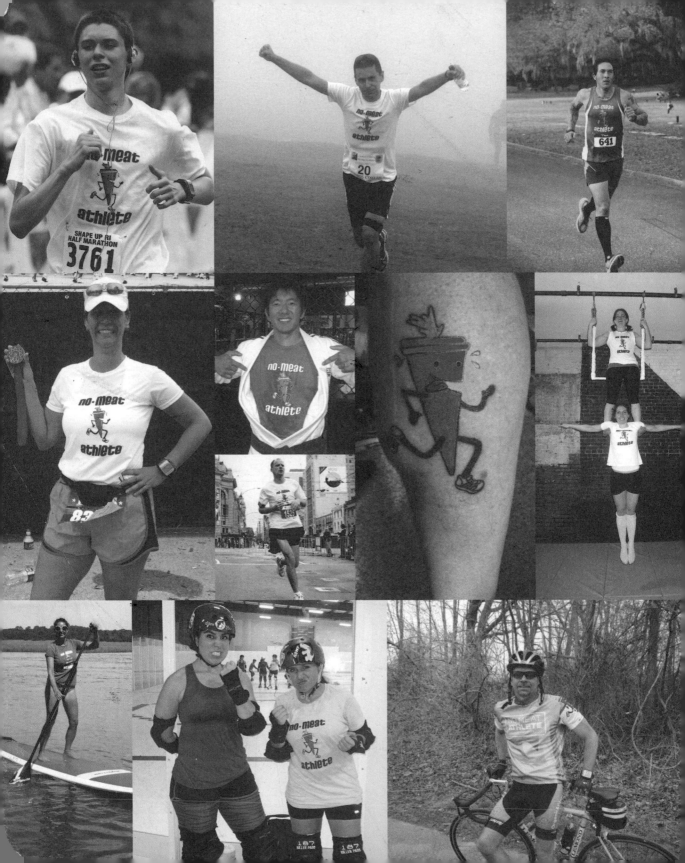